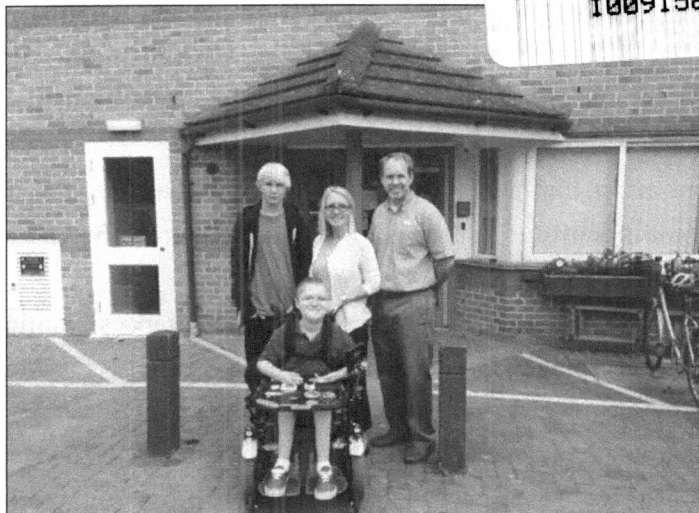

The Cottor Family visiting Helen House (Oxford, England) – July 2014

Thank You!

A project like Ryan House, and even this book about its creation, takes many, many people. Our family is humbled and so appreciative of our wonderful community, partners, and the scores of individuals who have shared the vision to bring a model like Helen House to Phoenix. This dedicated corps – the "village" it has taken to realize the dream of Ryan House – continues to work tirelessly to assure that Ryan House is sustained and available for those families most in need.

Our wish with this book was to capture in writing the magic of how stars aligned around our personal experiences and share a glimpse of how Ryan House developed. Our goal is to share why respite and palliative care is so important for families on this most difficult journey. In doing so, we hope to inspire other communities to champion something similar…after all, if it can be done in Phoenix, it can be done elsewhere as well. Let's have 100's of these houses in the United States soon!

A short book like this only skims the surface of the steadfast work that went into creating Ryan House. We have tried to feature major milestones and key moments from the history that were especially important to achieving success. As said, there have been so many people involved, we wish we could fill volumes to thank each and every one whose contribution has been important and valued.

There are a few people and organizations that must be mentioned by name, for it is truly due to their personal passion, commitment, and drive that Ryan House exists today.

First and foremost, we wish to thank Sister Frances Dominica, Founder and Trustee of Helen House, and Helen House itself. It is the world-class care that our family received at Helen House, the first children's hospice in the world, that inspired us to advocate for similar care in Arizona.

It is also with deepest thanks that we wish to recognize Judy and Bill Schubert. Judy was the driving force and wind in our sails. Our good fortune to connect with Judy, whose aptitude to immediately "get it" and willingness to embrace the project, was the best thing that could have ever happened for Ryan House. Together, Judy and Bill introduced possibilities for land, architects, construction, design and so much more. We wish every community finds and connects with its own "Judy and Bill Schubert."

Susan Levine was always there to catch us and propel us to the next level. She was literally the first formal conversation Holly had about the need for a pediatric palliative care home in Phoenix. From that moment on, Susan provided the wings to help us soar. Her vision, and willingness "to do whatever it takes" to make this project a reality is without question the reason Ryan House has an innovative and sustainable business model and something that we hope can be replicated in other communities.

We also wish to recognize and thank Linda Hunt. The land offer from her organization was the major milestone we needed to legitimize our team efforts, and put us on the map. Linda's belief in the mission of Ryan House was felt so strongly, not only by our group but throughout our community. She went above and beyond our wildest dreams to give Ryan House a home... "without any strings attached." There simply are no words to describe the highest gratitude for that gift to the community.

Rallying a community to come together for a project like this took entire organizations as well. We wish to take a moment and reflect on the original Founding Community Partner organizations, for which Ryan House is so grateful:

- The Board of Visitors
- Dignity Health St. Joseph's Hospital and Medical Center
- Hospice of the Valley
- The Junior League of Phoenix, Inc.
- Kitchell Contractors, Inc.
- Orcutt | Winslow Partnership
- St. Luke's Health Initiatives

Community Partners:

- Phoenix Children's Hospital
- IntraMedia Solutions, LLC

Along the project journey, we often paused to pinch ourselves and ask if this was really happening. It just seemed that the right people were coming together at the right time to create something very special. We thought it would be great to document this someday…and then one day, "someday" happened. We received a call from Excellence in Giving, a philanthropic advisory firm representing Mrs. Doris Lumsden. Mrs. Lumsden supported Ryan House while living in Arizona. Although she had moved out of state, Mrs. Lumsden wanted to help others learn about Ryan House and inspire them to do similar work. It is with heartfelt gratitude that we thank the Richard Lumsden Foundation for providing the launch funding for this book project, and the group at Excellence in Giving for connecting us with Mark Tabb to beautifully tell the story.

Finally, all of this work is done for the families we serve. We are so proud to share some of the amazing family stories in this book. At the time of publishing, Ryan House is celebrating its 5-year anniversary. Throughout those years, hundreds of children and their families have now become part of the "Ryan House family." We are grateful for those willing to share their very personal stories to help others understand why and how Ryan House impacts them. We wish we had volumes to share more.

In closing, we thank each and every supporter, from young children donating gifts in lieu of their own presents...to granting corporations, for their continued passion and commitment to Ryan House. Ryan House is a community project and it is our community that will sustain it. Our personal goal and wish was simply to bring a model like Helen House to Phoenix... nothing more, but also nothing less. Our community realized the unique need for word-class care and programs to embrace Arizona children and their families as they navigate life-limiting or end-of-life journeys.

Now...so can yours.

With deep appreciation,

The Cottor Family
Jonathan, Holly, Ethan, and Ryan

Ryan House
In the Heart of Phoenix

By Mark Tabb
With Holly and Jonathan Cottor

*"...no matter how long, or how short,
all lifetimes have beginnings, and endings,
and there is living in between."*[1]

---

1 From *Lifetimes* by Bryan Mellonie and Robert Ingpen

13 ISBN: 978-0-9905157-7-7 (paperback)

Cover features: Child Life Clinical Coordinator Kristen Bakalis w/ Hilary and Volunteer Terrence Swann w/ Hannah

Interior design: Debbi Stocco, mybookdesigner.com

Published by Ryan House
Printed in the USA

Table of Contents

Foreword

I first met the Cottor family at a breakfast to discuss a concept they hoped to bring to life in Phoenix. Ryan, their youngest son, had an illness that had introduced the Cottors to Helen House, a welcoming facility that provides respite and hospice care for children and their families in England.

I was so moved by the Cottors' passion and the need for such a facility in Phoenix, that I toured Helen House while visiting Oxford. There, I witnessed the impact the facility had on children and their families. This warm, cozy home was a happy place that fulfilled an important care niche. I was determined that St. Joseph's Hospital and Medical Center would make this type of care available to families in our area who have ill children and no help.

The visit provided inspiration to make "Ryan House" a reality in Phoenix. St. Joseph's had a piece of land that was perfect for such a project, and we were able to offer and pay for a 60-year lease to Ryan House for $1 a year. The magic continued as Ryan House was built.

Today, my office overlooks Ryan House. I am reminded daily of the importance of this facility and the wonderful services it provides to children and their families.

Linda Hunt
Sr. Vice President of Operations, Arizona
Dignity Health

Introduction

Party Time at Ryan House

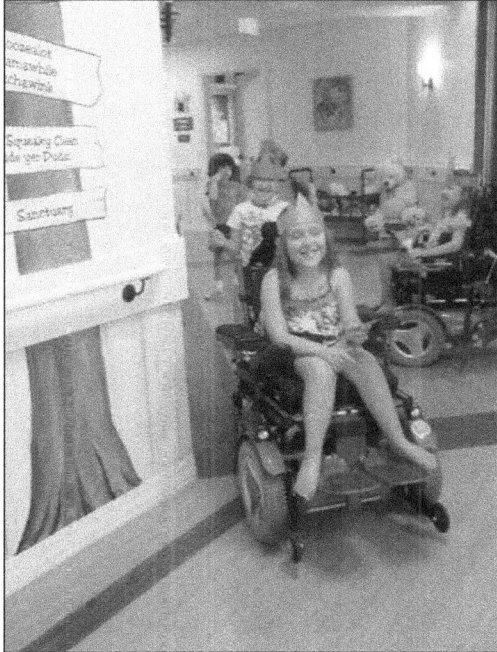

Madi at Ryan House

Madi is throwing a party. But then again, if Madi is in the house, a party will break out sooner rather than later. Madi loves parties, and she especially loves throwing them. If a career as a fashion designer doesn't work out for her some day, she'll probably become a party planner. It's not so much the planning she enjoys as it is being in charge. (And when Madi throws a party, she calls all the shots.) Watching Madi put her party plans into action, one gets the feeling that parties aren't the only time she's in charge. At home, she bosses around her six year old sister like any self-respecting big sister would. At least that's what Madi says. Her little sister isn't here to say any different. This is Madi's weekend free from her sister and free from her parents. Getting away from her parents is her favorite thing about coming to Ryan House; that and throwing parties.

Today Madi has a planning partner, Alissa. The two became buddies during one of their stays at Ryan House. Even though Alissa is three years younger than Madi, the two have a lot in common. For one, they both love parties. They also share a love of crafts, music, swimming and the Disney Channel. And they both have pink power chairs on which they fly up and down the halls of Ryan House. Both need the chairs because they also share the same life limiting condition where their muscles don't work the way most eight and eleven year old girls' muscles work. For reasons researchers do not yet understand, Madi and Alissa lack a gene which produces a protein essential to motor neurons. Without it, the neurons degenerate and eventually die. Most children born with the most severe form of this condition do not live to see their second birthday.

Watching Madi and Alissa in action, one would never guess their condition has such a grave prognosis. Outside of their chairs, they're just like all other preteen girls planning their next big event. Today's big event is the Mask Blast. Yesterday Madi threw a scarf party, but Alissa wasn't there to help. Instead, Madi had to rely on Ashley. Ashley works at Ryan House as a child life specialist. It's an important job with a long job description, but when Ashley arrives her job consists primarily of making sure Madi has everything she needs for her parties, and helping her pull them off. When Ashley noticed Madi's name on the guest list for the weekend, she stocked the Ryan House kitchen with fruit for Madi's fruit kabobs. She also bought a couple of boxes of cake mix. After all, you can't have a party without cake. The night before Alissa arrived, Ashley and Madi worked together in the kitchen baking and preparing for a weekend of partying. Madi helped stir a can of pumpkin into cake batter, although Ashley had to turn the crank on the can opener and lift up the can. Madi's muscles are too weak for those tasks.

There was enough cake left over from the scarf party for Mask Blast. That freed Madi and Alissa to spend most of their time in the art room making masks for all the guests to wear. The two girls made masquerade masks out of construction paper and attached popsicle sticks as handles. Every mask also received lots and lots of glitter. To a preteen girl, life demands glitter.

The girls needed help making their sparkly vision a reality, but that is not a problem at Ryan House. Mary was there to help. She worked the scissors to cut out the mask and fetched the varieties of markers and glitter Madi and Alissa needed to make each mask unique. Mary volunteers at Ryan House once or twice a month. Some days she reads to the children, or she pulls those who are not mobile through the halls in their wagons or pushes them along in their wheelchairs. Today she was on party mask making duty. She knows, as do all of the staff and guests, that Mask Blast was to be the social event of the season, at least until the party Madi plans to throw tomorrow.

While Madi and Alissa decorated the masks using markers and stickers, Kasia, a member of the staff care team, walked past pulling a little boy named Seven along in his wagon. Seven had nodded off, but he woke up when he heard the activity coming from the art room. Kasia brought him inside. Although Seven is not mobile and cannot speak, he has a way of letting people know what he wants. Today, he wanted to watch Madi and Alissa. Madi took his entrance in stride. Of course he wanted to be a part of getting ready for Mask Blast. Didn't everyone in the house?

A message is scrawled across the glass doors leading into the great room: "Mask Blast today at 2." The time will probably change. It often does for a Madi party. During her last visit, she threw a Hawaiian Party, complete with grass skirts. All the guests had to don the skirts and do the hula, including visiting football players from Phoenix's Arizona Rattlers Arena League team. Madi draped her skirt around her chair and danced by moving her chair back and forth while waving her other arm. She loves to dance. "If my legs worked, I would be a dancer," she says matter-of-factly without a tinge of self-pity. When you attend one of Madi's parties, you quickly get the impression that she doesn't waste a lot of time on self-pity, at least not while she's at Ryan House. There's too much for her to do here.

Promptly at 3:10, Mask Blast swings into motion. Madi and Alissa sit behind a table, handing cut masks to all the guests. Seven is there, as is another boy, Santana. Neither is mobile nor can communicate verbally, but that doesn't matter. Every child staying at Ryan House this weekend is invited. John, a retired engineer, dons the first mask. Brett comes in from the back office. He's the youngest and only male member of the office staff that handles the business side of Ryan House. His appearance makes Madi break out in a smile. "I have something for you," she calls to him. Brett knows the drill. He smiles back and steps into the great room ready to be humiliated. In his two years at Ryan House he's worn plenty of scarves and hats and costumes as part of the parties, which guests like Madi love to throw.

Jessica quietly slips in the back, her two year old daughter in tow. The two of them are not here for the party nor does Jessica have a child staying at the house, at least, she doesn't any more. Jessica stopped by Ryan House on this particular Friday afternoon to visit the memory garden just off the sanctuary room. This visit is very different from those she used to make. Not that long ago, as the parent of one of the children for whom Ryan House was built, Jessica used the house for respite. She can still see the smile that broke out on her little girl's face whenever they walked through these doors. Now the smile is a memory; one that Ryan House helps keep alive for her.

By 4:00 Mask Blast has run its course. Madi names Rachel (one of the nurses on staff) Queen while Brett is named King. Brett winning the honor of Mask Blast King is a bit of a surprise. Madi never names boys the king of her parties for one simple reason: "I don't like them," she says with a sly smile.

"But what about..." Ashley replies.

Madi quickly cuts her off. "I told you I don't like him," she says, her face turning multiple shades of red.

With Mask Blast in the history books, Madi and Alissa discuss what to do next. They have less than two days left together on their break from their parents and are determined to squeeze out as much fun as they can. If it weren't early September with an outside temperature hovering near 110°, they might have gone outside to the very wheelchair friendly playground. Instead, they opt for the indoor pool. Technically, the pool is known as the hydrotherapy room, but for girls like Madi and Alissa, the pool represents freedom. "I love the pool," Alissa says, "it's the only place my arms and legs work like they are supposed to."

Rachel suits up and joins them in the pool as does another staff member. It takes a while to change Madi and Alissa into their suits and slide their water wings on their arms to help them float. A special poolside mechanical chair lowers each girl down into the pool, then lifts them out again when the girls get bored with swimming and decide to go to the Story of Me Room to create music videos and movies with the state-of-the art multimedia equipment.

A couple of hours later, Madi and Alissa were hanging out next to the reception desk. Technically it's the care team center for charting and communications, but it doesn't look like one, at least not until you step to the other side and discover the monitors where they keep track of all the children in each of the house's eight bedrooms. But Madi and Alissa don't care about any of that. They were waiting for their next victims, and they didn't have to wait long. The moment Mark Tabb, an author of this book, walked out of the conference room that doubled as his office during his stay at Ryan House, Madi looked up at him with an evil, little grin. "It's time," she said.

"Time? For what?" he asked.

"You'll see," Madi replies. One of the nurses slid a rolling office chair out from behind the reception desk and placed it behind Madi's power chair. "Sit down and hold on," she instructed him. Mark did as he was told. The next thing he knew, he was flying down the hall, holding on for dear life as Madi flung her chair from side to side, trying to shake him free like a rodeo bull trying to lose a rider. He narrowly missed crashing into the walls, which only made Madi more determined to lose him. His left hand broke free, causing him to turn sharply to his right. Next thing he knew, his office chair was side by side with Madi, with his back to the direction they were going. "Well imagine meeting you here?" he said. Madi just smiled and made a sharp turn, sending his chair back around to the back.

After Mark's lap down the hall with Madi, Alissa looked at him and said, "I'm next. Hold on."

Parties in the great room and chair races down the hallway are part of the appeal of Ryan House for children like Madi and Alissa, but only part. What makes this place so special to children with life-threatening conditions goes beyond the fun they have, although fun is important. And it goes beyond the caring staff and the army of volunteers who make Ryan House possible. The children don't know or care about the fact that Ryan House is offered free of charge to families with children like Madi and Alissa. No, the real appeal of Ryan House to Madi and Alissa and Seven and Santana and all the rest of the children who have made this their home away from home is simply this: Here, they do not stand out because of their limitations. During their stays at Ryan House, these children feel wonderfully normal no matter what challenges they may face on a daily basis and no matter what their long term prognosis may be. This is a place where children who probably will not live to see adulthood can come and play away from mom and dad and feel like typical children. This is also a place where those same children and their families come as those conditions or diseases reach their ultimate conclusion.

Madi does not know how fortunate she is to live in the greater Phoenix area, for Ryan House is one of only two places like it in the entire United States of America. It might not exist at all if not for another child whose parents were told he had the same condition as Madi when he was only eight months old.

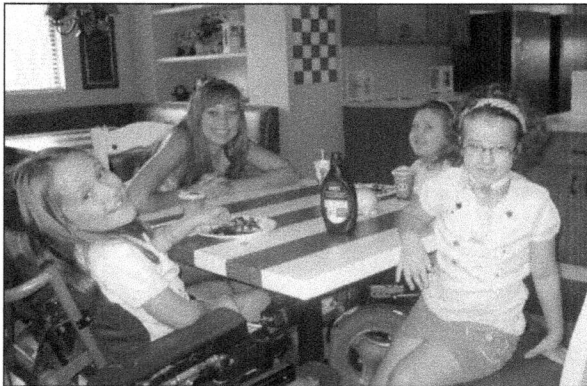

Madi, Destiny, and Cloey with a volunteer at Ryan House

Section One: A Dream Born Out of a Nightmare

Chapter One

Something's Not Right

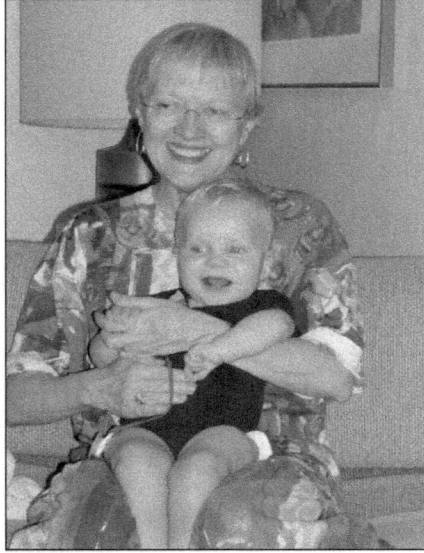

Nana (Jonathan's mom, Sharon) and Ryan

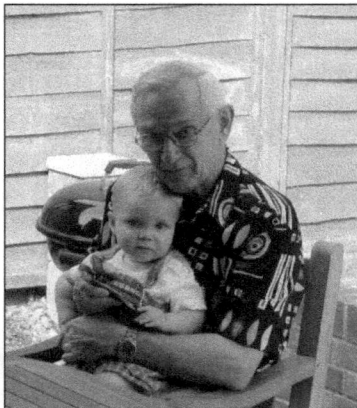

Grandpa (Jonathan's dad, Bob) and Ryan

A WAVE OF NAUSEA WASHED over Holly as she watched her husband's parents hold their newest grandchild for the first time since shortly after he was born. Although she and Jonathan had several conversations lately about Ryan not yet rolling over or crawling or sitting up on his own like most eight month old babies, the two of them always found a way to explain away his slow progress. "He's a late bloomer...He's just a little lazy...He isn't behind, it just seems that way compared to his big brother..." However, the looks on Bob and Sharon Cottor's faces told her that all her worst fears were about to be confirmed.

Holly first suspected something was not right with her newborn son when he did not grip his big brother Ethan's finger as Ethan stroked Ryan's palm. Their Grammy, Holly's grandmother, had said, "Tell Ethan that that's how his baby brother will say 'I love you!'" He'll grab on tight to your finger. Later, he'll want to sit by you to tell you he loves you. Then he'll crawl to you and finally walk over next to you to tell you he loves you..." But, Ryan never did grab hold of Ethan or crawl over toward him.

Even so, Holly and Jonathan chalked up their fears to nothing more than the normal paranoia every parent of a newborn feels when they jump to the conclusion that a little cough is the onset of pneumonia. Even the medical professionals who saw Ryan[2] didn't seem overly alarmed. "Every child develops in his or her own time," Holly and Jonathan heard over and over. When Ryan failed to sit up at six months of age, a general practitioner prescribed a physical therapy evaluation. However, the therapist's office had a long wait list and no one pushed to move Ryan to the front of it. Holly took that to mean they thought Ryan would probably start sitting on his own sooner rather than later.

One day I will walk into his room and find him sitting and pulling up and rolling over and crawling around his crib, all in the same day, Holly told herself over and over. After all, he was well ahead of the curve in all other aspects of his development. He was the happiest, easiest and most enjoyable baby Holly could ever hope for.

---

2 In England, children don't see a pediatrician unless an issue surfaces. Otherwise, children receive care through the local Health Centre which includes Health Visitors who come to your home.

Watching Bob and Sharon exchange a look after Sharon passed Ryan over to Bob told Holly she needed to prepare herself for a new reality.

But thoughts of the worst kept flooding over her. Try as she might, Holly could not convince herself that she was witnessing nothing more than travel fatigue and jet lag. "Where is our little lovebug?" Sharon crooned when she and Bob first walked into what they referred to as "the dollhouse" – Holly and Jonathan's home in Harefield, on the outskirts of London. She didn't look tired. If anything, playing with Ethan on the drive from the airport had reenergized Nana and Grandpa. It was, after all, the reason Bob and Sharon had traveled more than 5,200 miles. Sure, they wanted to see Holly and Jonathan, but more than anything, they wanted to play with their grandsons.

She pushed the thoughts out of her head the best she could. *They're just tired*, she thought. *The flight from Phoenix to England wears anyone out! Don't be paranoid. Don't overreact. Don't assume the worst.*

Bob and Sharon's excitement evaporated the moment Holly placed Ryan in Sharon's arms. Tears welled up in Sharon's eyes and they did not appear to Holly to be tears of joy. Sharon didn't hold Ryan long, not nearly as long as Holly thought she would. Holly had joked with Jonathan about how the two of them wouldn't get to hold their sons during the entire two weeks of Jonathan's parents' visit. Now Sharon seemed eager to hand Ryan off to her husband. *Bob's a doctor and a child psychiatrist. Is that why she handed him over so fast?* Holly wondered. *Does she want an expert's opinion?*

As Grandpa spent some time with Ryan on the couch, Holly and Sharon stepped into the kitchen. Holly swallowed hard. *Just say it!* she thought, but the words did not want to come out. Standing in the kitchen, Holly understood that she stood on a precipice she did not want to cross. The moment she asked the question welling up inside of her, she feared nothing would ever be the same. *He's just a late bloomer,* she told herself one last time before asking, "Is something wrong?"

"I am so sorry, Holly. We have to find a doctor for Ryan." Sharon's voice cracked. A very caring, compassionate and educated woman who'd spent her career working with at-risk children as a family therapist, she'd had conversations like this with mothers before, but never with her daughter-of-the-heart, never discussing one of her own grandchildren. Sharon did not know exactly what was going on, but she suspected the diagnosis was not going to be good.

Holly began to weep. "Did I do something wrong?" she asked. "What could I have done to cause this? Could I have hurt him somehow?" Having asked her own mom the same questions by phone just a couple of months earlier, these questions still lingered in her mind.

"No, no, no, Holly," Sharon comforted as she wrapped her arms around Holly. "You haven't done anything wrong. You didn't cause this. How could you? You've been a great mother."

"But what if I did something before he was born that harmed him? What if I bounced him too enthusiastically on my lap while singing and playing with him? I don't know how I can live with myself if I did this to my baby."

"I don't know for sure, but I suspect whatever is causing this had nothing to do with you," Sharon said as she tried to reassure Holly. The two women stood in the kitchen for a very long time, holding onto one another, weeping. Bob and Jonathan joined them. The line had been crossed. There was no going back.

Family friends, also general practitioners, recommended a nearby Developmental Pediatrician. A couple of days later, Holly, Jonathan and his father, Bob, took Ryan to an appointment while Sharon stayed home with Ethan. Unlike their visit for Ryan's six month check-up, the Developmental Pediatrician validated their concerns. He examined Ryan thoroughly and then looked carefully in Ryan's mouth. "I notice Ryan has something called 'fasciculations,' a kind of muscle twitch. These twitches can indicate that nerves are having difficulty sending signals to muscles. I can't be certain without testing, but I think Ryan has something called Spinal Muscular Atrophy (SMA). I'd like to refer you to a neurologist at Hammersmith Hospital, where they can confirm a diagnosis with genetic testing."

"Okay," Holly said. Now her worst fears had a name, although she did not know anything about it.

That night, Holly, Jonathan and Bob scoured the internet for anything and everything remotely related to SMA. "Spinal Muscular Atrophy (SMA) is an inherited neuromuscular condition that particularly affects nerve cells that originate in the spinal cord," they read on a website. "SMA is a rare disease that affects approximately 1 in 6,000 babies...a recessive genetic disorder... About 1 in 40 of us is a carrier... four main types of SMA – Types 1, 2 and 3 appear in childhood, while Type 4 affects adults." Reading that SMA is a genetic disorder alleviated part of Holly's guilt that she'd done something to hurt Ryan. Even so, she could not shake the feeling that she had somehow failed to protect her baby. Most parents who live through hearing a potentially life limiting diagnosis for their children wrestle with the same feelings, no matter how many times physicians and therapists reassure them that they've done nothing wrong.

Holly and Jonathan eventually headed off to bed while Bob continued his research late into the night. The next morning he reported all he'd learned. "From what I'm learning, this can be very serious. Ryan clearly doesn't have Type 4, but I'm hopeful he has the mild form of SMA, maybe type 3. That would mean that Ryan would live with a life-changing disability, but he could still have a fairly normal lifespan."

"So that's what we hope for, worst case scenario type 3, best case type 4," Jonathan said.

"Type 4 only affects adults," Bob corrected him.

"So Type 3 then," Jonathan said.

"But what if..." Holly said.

"Then we deal with the hand we're dealt. But let's not worry about what ifs until we have to," Jonathan said.

"I hope that you are able to see the neurologist soon so that you can learn exactly what Ryan will be living with, what we will all be living with. Childhood disabilities have an impact on everyone in the family," Sharon added.

Later that month, Holly and Jonathan carried Ryan into Hammersmith Hospital with trepidation, knowing that genetic testing would verify the severity of his condition. "Tell me what you understand about SMA," the physician professor asked. After they recited what they'd learned about the different types and their hopes that Ryan would have a more mild form, the neurologist explained. "We won't know for certain which type Ryan has until all the tests are done. Only then can I give you a realistic long-term prognosis for your son. I'll see you again once results have come back."

Ryan endured a muscle biopsy, blood draws for genetic tests, and an EKG along with physical therapy evaluations. Holly and Jonathan watched, looking for answers in the reaction of the doctors and therapists to Ryan's responses, but they weren't sure what they were looking for. Although they knew Ryan's diagnosis, they weren't sure what it meant or what, if any, treatments were available. At this point, all they had were questions, with the biggest one being: What does the future hold for Ryan?

Two days after Ryan's tests at Hammersmith Hospital, Holly got up early on a Saturday morning to go for a run. The house was quiet. No one had yet stirred, which was unusual. Quiet moments are hard to find with two small children. Holly had spent most of the previous evening doing what she did with most of her spare time: searching the internet for information about SMA. She had to understand what her young son was up against. After reading so much information the night before, most of it depressing, she had to get out and do something to clear her mind. And nothing clears the mind like an early morning run.

As she slipped on her running shoes, she noticed an envelope from Hammersmith had been slipped through the mail slot in the door. Her heart sank. She started to tug on the edge to open it, but hesitated. She took a deep breath and let it out slowly. "Okay, so this is it," she said. Carefully, she tore open the envelope and pulled out the letter inside. On top, just under the Hammersmith masthead, she saw Ryan's name and birth date. Beside it, in letters that lunged at her off the page, she read, "Diagnosis: Type I, SMA."

Holly dropped the letter, laced up her shoes, and ran out the door. She took off, running hard through the streets. Tears rolled down her cheeks as she ran faster and faster, trying to get as far as fast as she could from the letter lying on her living room floor. A heavy set, middle aged woman walked out of her house and stared as Holly ran by. *She must think I'm a crazy American running through the village like this* Holly thought to herself. She kept running and running until she could not go any further. Her legs gave way.

Holly fell to the ground, sobbing, unable to move. When she finally returned home, Jonathan was sitting in the living room, letter in hand. "You saw this already?" he asked.

"Yeah."

He paused. "So now I guess we wait for the doctor to explain all this so we'll know exactly what we're dealing with." He didn't come out and say it, but Holly sensed her husband still held onto the hope, albeit a faint hope, that the report didn't tell the whole story and that the genetic test would show Ryan as a Type 2 at the worst.

"I guess so," she said. Neither said anything else for what felt like a very long time.

Three weeks later, on Valentine's Day, the two of them sat down in the neurologist's office, listening as he explained the test results. "We grade these on a continuum. Even within the three types of SMA in childhood, there are levels of severity with varying prognoses. We estimate that Ryan is somewhere between 1.9–2.1."

Jonathan asked, "So what exactly does that mean?"

"It means your son is possibly a strong type 1 or a weak type 2. It also means his long-term prognosis is poor. Up to eighty percent of children with the most severe form of SMA do not survive to their second birthday."

Holly struggled to maintain her composure. She already knew these statistics from researching SMA on the internet. However, it is one thing to read words on a web page and quite another to listen to a doctor say them about your son.

"Does Ryan have the most severe form?" Jonathan asked.

The neurologist paused, choosing his words very carefully. "Your son has a life shortening condition for which there is no treatment or cure. How long will he live? I cannot say for sure. No one can. All I can tell you is that statistically, eighty percent of children with Type 1 SMA do not survive to the age of two. I'm very sorry to have to tell you this."

Holly and Jonathan clutched one another's hands, their minds reeling. "So what are we supposed to do now?" Jonathan finally asked.

"The two of you need to discuss the quality of life you would like Ryan to have; that is, do you want him to live at all costs, even if it means special equipment is keeping him alive?"

"Special equipment?" Holly asked.

"Ventilators, G-tubes[3], that sort of thing. Many children with SMA reach a point where they cannot survive without them. Or would you prefer that he not live with invasive procedures and equipment, even though he may not live as long? These are choices only the two of you can make, and you will need to make them together. For now, take him home. Love him. Enjoy the time you have with your son."

Jonathan and Holly looked at one another without saying a word. The thin hope to which they both clung was yanked from their hands.

"Now what?" Jonathan sobbed as they left. "Now what?"

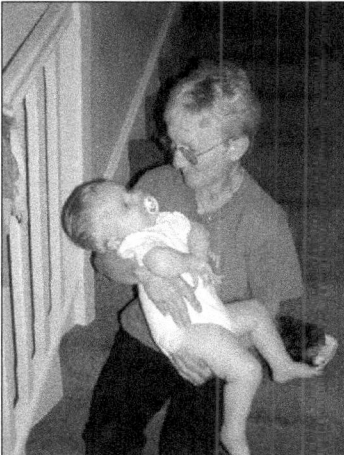

Abuelita (Holly's mom, Judi)
with Ryan

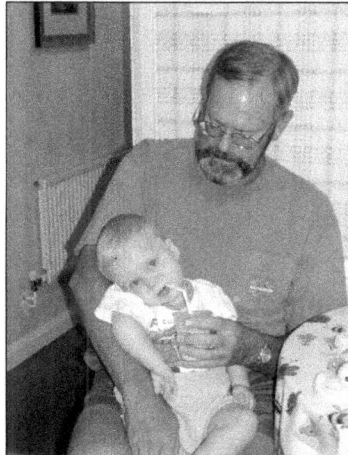

Papa (Holly's dad, Budd)
with Ryan

---

3 Gastrostomy tube, aka a feeding tube.

Chapter Two

A House Called Helen

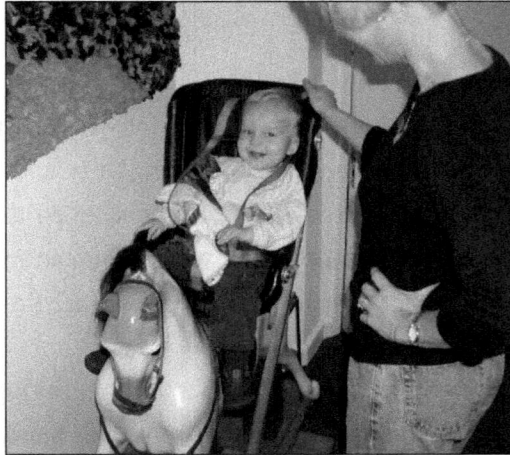

Holly and Ryan visit Helen House

"WE NEED TO TALK."

"I know, but not now. I can hardly hold my eyes open."

Jonathan let out a long sigh. "When, then?"

"I don't know. Maybe the day after Ryan sleeps through the night," Holly said with a little laugh. She got up off the sofa and headed toward their bedroom.

"This isn't funny."

Holly spun around and shot a look that said more than she wanted. "What do you want me to say? Sure, now's a great time to talk about what 'nature taking its course' is going to look like!"

"We have to talk about it at some time." Jonathan tried to hide his agitation. He reminded himself that they were both exhausted. When Ryan was born, they both knew they were in for a lot of sleepless nights. But neither of them expected the sleepless nights to go on indefinitely. Ryan's SMA left him unable to reposition himself during the night, which caused him to become very uncomfortable every hour or two. His discomfort would wake him up and he then would cry until someone came and moved him. Going through this same routine night after night without end meant that Jonathan and Holly were both seriously sleep-deprived.

"We have talked, and we both agree: No vents. No G-tubes. No extreme measures." She leaned over against the wall, as if standing required more energy than her body could produce, which was not far from the truth. On weeknights, Holly got up with Ryan at least four times each night. Usually more. Then she had to get up early every morning to meet the needs of a very active almost four year old whose motor never seemed to stop while also doing everything for Ryan that she had to do when he was first born; all with very little outside help since every close family member lived on the other side of the Atlantic. Throw in teaching at a local school, trying to be a good wife and taking care of the household needs, and Holly was about to give up. Jonathan got up with Ryan on weekends to give her a little extra sleep, but she never caught up. The past year had worn out both of them with no end in sight.

"But..." Jonathan added, then stopped. Holly's slumped shoulders and half opened eyes told him to save his breath. "We'll...we'll talk later."

"Thank you," Holly replied. She turned back toward the bedroom. "Are you coming to bed?"

"Not yet. I have some work I need to finish before tomorrow," Jonathan said. Holly stumbled down the hallway as he sat down at his desk. He opened his laptop to find the files he needed to look over, but his heart wasn't in it. Work could wait. He really did need to talk, badly. Yet, aside from Holly, he had no one in his life who could possibly understand what he was going through. Every day co-workers asked how Ryan was doing, and every day he gave the same simple answer. "He's okay." No one really wanted to hear more than that, and Jonathan didn't know what he would say if he was honest with any of them.

The truth was, he didn't really know how Ryan was doing. The doctors' prognosis was bad, horrible really, yet Jonathan had no clue what to expect as the condition wore on. *Eighty percent of children with Type 1 SMA don't survive to their second birthday* he was told, which meant Ryan only had a twenty percent chance of surviving the next twelve months. *We'll let nature take its course*, they had agreed. The decision tore them both up, but they really had no other choice. Ryan's condition could not be cured. Nature was going to take its course with or without their consent. *But what does that really mean?* he wondered. *Will Ryan slowly deteriorate or will he take a sudden turn for the worse and die?* The thought of losing his young son made Jonathan ill. He'd only faced death close up one time and that was with a grandfather suffering from Alzheimer's. Now he found he had to prepare himself for every parent's worst nightmare. Old men who've lived full lives and now find themselves suffering a cruel and incurable disease die. Not children, and especially not babies.

But there was more to it than simply the dread of losing a child. Jonathan's biggest fear was not Ryan dying, since he knew that was inevitable, but the fear that Ryan might die while he was alone with him. *What if he dies on my watch...?* gnawed at him. He could not relax as a father and truly enjoy his son. And he certainly did not want Holly to leave him at home alone with Ryan. Sure, he could care for Ryan. He could change his diapers and feed him and do everything a dad needs to do. But the "what ifs" terrified him. *What if Ryan chokes on a Cheerio? What if he stops breathing? What if he suddenly dies with me? Would that be nature taking its course, or me failing to do my job as his dad?*

Jonathan stared at his computer screen, clicking here and there with his mouse, accomplishing nothing for over an hour. He decided to close up shop when he heard Ryan cry. "It's going to be another long night," he said as he closed his laptop and headed toward Ryan's room.

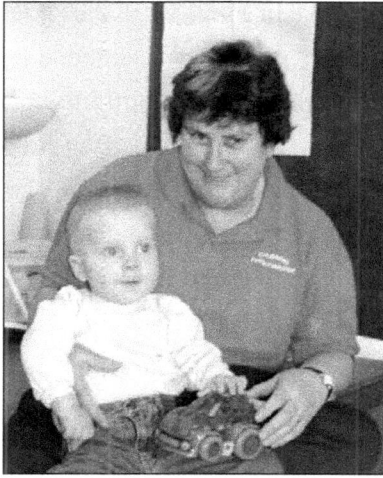

Ann with Ryan

The next morning Holly, bleary eyed and on edge, took Ryan in for his regular physical therapy appointment. "How are you doing this morning, Holly?" Ann, the physiotherapist, asked as she worked with Ryan on a mat on the floor.

Holly tried to force out the lie of *Fine, just fine*, but she could not do that again. "Honestly? Not so good." Holly tried to hold herself together, but tears began to flow. That one honest answer threatened to break the dam and allow a torrent of honest emotion to come pouring out. She fought the urge to tell Ann that she was tired, depressed, and angry. Instead, she bit her lip and said, "I'm sorry. I shouldn't be doing this."

"What? Being human? Why would you apologize for that? Dealing with your son's condition will wear even the strongest souls down." Ann got up from the floor and returned with a small brochure. "There's a place not far from here called Helen House, a children's hospice, that's for families like yours. I've heard from other families that it's really lovely. They're set up there to care for your son, to give you and your husband a bit of a respite."

Holly took the brochure and turned it over in her hand. The photo on the front showed a warm, inviting home. She opened it and read "Helen House is a bright, comfortable home-away-from-home for children from birth to eighteen years old with life-shortening conditions." Photos of special needs children, smiling and laughing, were sprinkled across the inside. As she glanced through the lines of text one sentence leapt off the page at her: "When a child or young adult has a life limiting condition, everyone in the family is affected." *What an understatement* she said to herself and kept reading. "Coming to terms with a new diagnosis, or a family member's changing condition, can create many challenges and families can feel overwhelmed by the choices and decisions they have to make." *Overwhelmed* was one word for what she was feeling. *Exhausted, at the end of her rope, not sure how she was going to face another day yet knowing she had no other choice* were other words she might have used. However one put it, clearly Helen House understood what they were going through. The brochure went on to describe the services Helen House offered to both the children with life-shortening conditions and their families. Both sounded very appealing.

"Can I keep this?" she asked.

"Of course," Ann replied. "Please, you and Jonathan should consider phoning to book an appointment to visit and have a look around. You need some rest and Helen House can help you."

Holly let out a little sigh. "That sounds nice. But, is it expensive to stay there?"

"There's no charge for the families," Ann said. "Conditions like your son's strike rich families and poor and those in the middle. Helen House is available at no charge to any family that needs its services."

"Wow. How can they do that?" Holly asked.

"Through donations. Many people here in the UK believe in the mission of Helen House and other children's hospices and give generously to make the care possible."

"Jonathan and I will have a look," she said as she stood to leave. She dropped the brochure into her purse, picked up Ryan and left.

On her trip home, she kept thinking about the photos of the children and the thought of actually getting a brief break from the demands of caring for her son. For a moment she fantasized about how good more than an hour or two of uninterrupted sleep would feel. But, Ann had said one thing that kept pulling Holly back into her reality. "A children's *hospice*," she said out loud to no one. *Hospice. Hospice is who you call in when someone is dying and you've given up hope. Hospice means you stop all treatment and just sit back and wait for the end to come. Hospice is waving the white flag. For Ryan? He's not dying. Why would we go to a hospice?*

Even with her hesitations, she showed the Helen House brochure to Jonathan later that evening and told him how Ann described it. "It can't hurt to visit," he said. "It sounds like just the thing we need."

"I don't know," she said. "I'm not sure I'm ready."

"For a break?"

"No. For hospice."

Over the next few weeks, Holly and Jonathan continued to switch off caring for Ryan during the night. Friends told them they needed to implement tough love with the little guy. "It's not the end of the world if he cries a little," they were told over and over. "Just let him cry and eventually he will go back to sleep on his own. He has the two of you trained to come running whenever he lets out the slightest peep. Show him some tough love for a night or two and he'll start sleeping through the night all on his own."

"But he can't turn himself," they replied. "That's why he cries."

"Lots of people sleep in one position all night long. It won't hurt him to learn to do the same."

Holly and Jonathan tried the tough love approach one night. Shortly after midnight, Ryan started crying, but the two of them stayed put. He cried louder and louder. They tried to ignore him. His cries grew more intense. Jonathan let out a long sigh. "I can't imagine how uncomfortable he has to be right now. Can we really do this?"

Holly began to weep softly. "I don't know."

"I mean," Jonathan said, "it's not his fault he can't move himself." He didn't come out and say it but to Holly the meaning was clear. Both felt guilty about passing down defective genes that caused Ryan's condition.

"No, it's not," Holly replied.

The two of them fought off the urge to go into Ryan's room that night, but they didn't sleep. Nor did they the next night. Finally, by night three, they abandoned tough love and went back to taking turns turning him over.

The mounting weeks of sleep deprivation led to a phone call to Helen House and a tour of the facilities. Jonathan could not get away from work for the tour, which did not matter to the two of them. "If you like it, so will I," he told her.

This is not what I expected was Holly's first thought as she walked into Helen House. While the house had that distinctive British no-nonsense feel, every room was bright and inviting. The eight bedrooms felt like children's bedrooms complete with teddy bears and toys sprinkled about. Each one had a large window that looked out on the green trees and blooming flowers of the central garden area. But what really impressed Holly was what she did not find in the bedrooms. Even though Ryan was only a year old, the Cottors had already spent enough time in doctor's offices and hospitals that Ryan bristled at anything that looked or smelled clinical. And she did as well. But walking through the rooms of Helen House she felt like she was at home. She didn't even recognize the doctors and nurses she was told were on staff. Everyone wore casual clothes, not scrubs.

Walking down the hall, Holly heard laughter coming from the dining room. Pausing, she noticed two families sharing a meal together. Further down the hall, a woman sat on the floor of the sensory room with a non-verbal little girl on her lap. The lights and images flashing from the ceiling projector to the floor that doubled as a screen captured the girl's attention in a way that made it clear she was enjoying herself. She wasn't alone. The worker, a middle aged woman, had a big grin on her face. Holly could tell the worker genuinely cared for this child.

An art room was just down the hallway. Holly poked her head in the door for a look around. Artwork adorned the walls, each clearly the handiwork of a child. Multicolored cabinets stood along a far wall with stacks of paper and a bin of markers sitting on the countertop. Two volunteers sat at the table next to a child in a wheelchair. Paint stains splashed across the tablecloth, yet that didn't make the room seem unkempt. If anything, the splotches of paint made the room feel authentic, like a dining room table in a home filled with children with big imaginations.

At the end of her tour, the staff politely answered Holly's questions. Before she left, the House manager handed Holly another brochure filled with information about how to schedule a stay. "We have four family flats available. Many families like to stay in the house to be near their children. But you don't have to stay here. Some of our children actually seem to prefer it when mum and dad go away and give them some space. Sort of like a trip to gran's house," the manager said.

Holly came away from her visit impressed, but something still bothered her. While touring the children's bedrooms her guide said, "We have eight rooms total. Six are always available for respite, but we normally keep the two on the end set aside for unplanned stays."

"Unplanned?" Holly replied.

"Yes. When a child is dying. These things often come quickly and unannounced. We keep rooms set aside for these families."

Of course, Holly thought. *That's why they call it a children's hospice. It's a place where children come to die.*

Holly politely thanked the staff for taking time to show her around, but made up her mind that Helen House was not for her family. She and Jonathan kept on with their regular routine, doing their best to push themselves as long as they could without giving out, each one trying to convince themselves that they could do this. "What choice do we have?" Holly said to her husband more than once. Yet, with each passing day, the two of them could feel their very limited internal resources depleting. Though neither wanted to admit it, they both knew they were near the limit of what they could endure.

One too many sleepless nights finally pushed Holly to pick up the phone and schedule a stay at Helen House. The idea of going to a hospice still struck her as just wrong, but she did not know where else to turn for a break. If she didn't get one soon, she knew both she and Jonathan would crack under the pressure.

Not long after checking into Helen House for the first time, Jonathan and Holly found themselves sitting across from another couple in the dining room. As conversations between parents always go, the talk soon turned to their children. "Our daughters love it here," the mom said.

"Do you always bring your other children with you when you stay?" Holly asked.

"We don't always stay here, but our daughters do. We have three who come here on a regular basis," the dad said.

Jonathan did not immediately catch the dad's inference. "So the siblings can stay overnight as well even without the two of you?" he asked.

"No. We have three daughters with life shortening conditions," the dad said. "They have Late Infantile Batten's disease. Are you familiar with it?"

Holly's heart jumped into her throat. *Three?! All three children have the same terminal condition.* She fought back tears. All these months she'd felt very, very alone in her struggle with her son's illness. Compared to this mom and dad sitting across from her, her struggles now seemed very small.

"Our younger son has SMA," Holly said, her voice cracking.

"Then you know..."

"I'm beginning to think I don't," Holly said. She felt embarrassed for feeling so tired from dealing with one child with a life threatening condition while the couple in front of her lived out her life three times over. "And... they...your daughters, are all staying here this weekend?" she asked.

"Not exactly," the dad said. "We're here for one of the rooms at the end of the hall. Our oldest daughter has taken a turn and is dying." Both Holly and Jonathan were more than a little surprised at the way in which this father shared this news. He spoke with a tone neither filled with grief nor cold. *He's at peace with what is happening*, Holly suddenly realized. *This is what nature taking its course looks like.*

For the next several minutes, the two couples talked, not as strangers who had just met, but with a warmth and familiarity of those who share an uncommon bond. For the first time, the Cottors were able to talk about the death of a child and not feel as if they'd broken some taboo by bringing up the subject. This couple, these strangers only a few minutes earlier, had a profound grasp on the fact that dying is a part of living, even for a child. Rather than hide from death, they embraced this stage of their daughter's life just as they had all those that had come before. To both Jonathan and Holly, the couple's outlook just felt natural.

The next morning, after a night of real, uninterrupted sleep, Jonathan and Holly found themselves next to one of Helen House's doctors in a quiet area set up for adults. Because Helen House is open to all people regardless of their religious beliefs, or lack of them, they do not have a formal chapel. Instead, this space provides a quiet place for prayer or meditation for anyone and everyone. It also gives parents a quiet place where they can escape the noise and activity of a house filled with children.

After a round of brief small talk, Jonathan finally asked the question that had gnawed at him since they'd first received Ryan's prognosis. "What does nature taking its course actually mean?"

The doctor smiled. "What exactly do you want to know?"

"We were told that our son only has a twenty percent chance of living to the age of two. He's not far from that now. Does that mean he's just going to suddenly stop breathing? How will I know when he's moving toward death?"

"You will know. His body won't suddenly give out in a matter of minutes or even days. You will observe changes over time that will give you a sense that he's getting weaker and death may be nearing."

"So he won't just go all of the sudden?" Jonathan asked, feeling a little silly for asking, but needing to know.

"No," the doctor said. "It won't be like that at all."

"Whew, that's a relief," Jonathan said. "I feel a little guilty for saying it, but since the day we got his diagnosis, I've been afraid to be alone with him."

"You have?" Holly said.

"Yes!" Jonathan said. "I was afraid that he would die on my watch and everyone would wonder why I didn't do more."

"No one would think that, Jonathan," Holly said.

"I would," he replied. Then, turning to the doctor, Jonathan asked, "Do you mind if I ask you another question that may seem obvious but it isn't to me?"

"Sure, go ahead," the doctor said.

"Holly and I agree that the best thing for our son is not to take wild, extreme measures to extend his life a short time at the cost of giving him real quality of life. So does that mean I should never call 9-9-9 (the British equivalent of 911)? What if Ryan chokes on a Cheerio? Do I let him choke or do I do something?"

"Jonathan!" Holly said.

He shrugged his shoulders. "I'm being honest here. I need someone to tell me what to do. They didn't cover this in *What to Expect When You're Expecting.*"

The doctor chuckled. "If he chokes on a Cheerio, you clear out the Cheerio, and if he needs more help, you get him more help. What the two of you have decided to do for your son is called palliative care. That means you focus on care that will give him the best quality of life possible by treating the symptoms and conditions that cause him pain and discomfort, while also doing all you can to help him live as full of a life as he can during the time he has. None of us have any guarantees about tomorrow. Palliative care operates on the premise that instead of focusing on squeezing out as many days as possible, we make the most of the time that we have."

Tears began to stream down Jonathan's face. He felt like a huge weight had just been lifted off his shoulders. Now, for the first time, he felt free to be a dad to his Ryan without carrying around the fear of what might happen. "That's what I want for my son."

"I know it is," the doctor said. "I know it is."

After that conversation, Holly and Jonathan spent the rest of their day focusing their full attention on Ethan while the Helen House staff took care of Ryan. By the time they left to return home they only had one regret – they wished they'd scheduled a stay at Helen House much, much sooner. They would not make that mistake again.

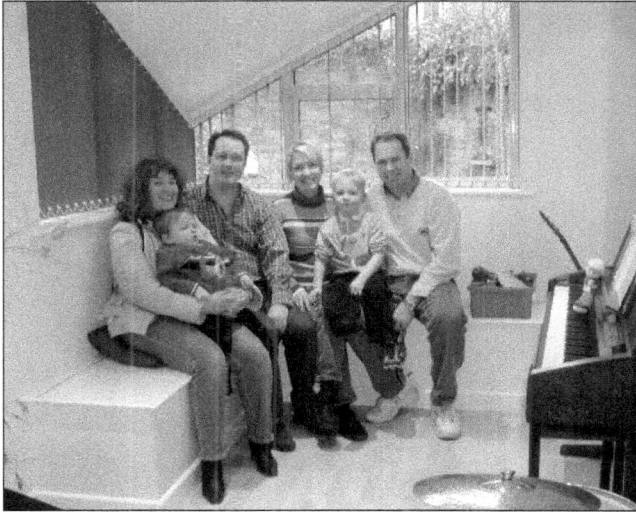

Holly, Jonathan, Ethan (right side) with friends
in the music room at Helen House

Anna and Caroline

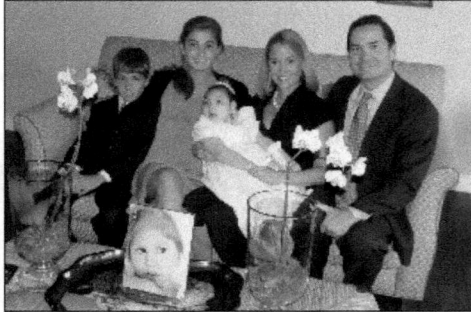

The Pierson Family

Anna's diagnosis came at a much earlier age than Caroline's.

With Caroline, no one suspected anything was wrong until her two month checkup. Up until then, she'd been a good, easy to care for baby. Looking back, her parents, Jim and Karrie, realized she was maybe too easy to care for. But, at the time they just chalked it up to finally knowing what they were doing. Caroline was their third child in six years. They dove into the parent pool with their daughter, Kat, and again two years later with their son, Joe. By the time Caroline came along they felt they had this baby thing down to a science. Karrie's pregnancy had been textbook as were her labor and delivery. Her doctors released her twenty four hours after Caroline's birth and sent them on their way. Nothing looked out of the ordinary.

However, something seemed amiss during a routine well baby checkup at two months. The pediatrician could not find a soft spot on Caroline's skull when he measured her head circumference. Nor could he feel any of the five sutures in her skull that allow the head to expand as the brain grows. "They're probably fused," he explained, which will prevent her brain from growing. However, since she is so young, surgery can probably correct it."

A few days later Jim and Karrie soon found themselves in the office of a neurosurgeon, expecting to hear him describe the operation Caroline would need. "Luckily they caught it early," Jim reassured Karrie on their way into his office. "We can do this."

The neurosurgeon walked in, x-rays in hand. "Okay, here's what we're looking at," he said as he entered. He quickly arranged the x-rays on the viewer on the wall, flipped on the light illuminating them, and announced with a very matter of fact tone, "I can't fix this. The sutures between her skull plates are fine. The problem is her brain is so small it can't push them out. It stopped growing at around twenty weeks gestation. It's really the worst outcome possible. I don't think her brain is developed enough to sustain her life for her first year."

Jim and Karrie looked at one another in shock. Neither could believe what they just heard. Finally Jim was able to say, "So our daughter is dying?"

"Basically, yes," the doctor said without a tinge of empathy. "It's really a grave prognosis without a course of treatment to correct it."

"What...uh...I uh, mean, uh what caused this?" Karrie stammered.

"That's a bit of a mystery," the doctor said. "Could have been any number of things. Something might have happened to you when you were pregnant that triggered it."

Karrie's mind raced back to the first half of her pregnancy. She'd been hospitalized with pneumonia and a high fever. The nurses had to pack her body in ice to bring her temperature down. "Could a high fever have done this?" she asked, trembling.

"That's possible but we can't know for sure," he said. "Sometimes these things just happen."

For the next few years Karrie carried the guilt that she had somehow harmed her precious little girl before her child was even born. If the high fever caused Caroline's brain to stop developing, that only meant Karrie should have sought help earlier. "Why did I wait so long to go to the hospital?" she tortured herself over and over. But it wasn't just the fever. Had she had something to eat or drink she shouldn't have? They say pregnant mothers should avoid coffee.

Did she? She could not say for sure. There was also that day about half way through her pregnancy when she volunteered at her older daughter's preschool. One of the children on the playground had barreled into her, nearly knocking her over. Could that have caused Caroline's condition?

With so many questions and no answers, Karrie took every precaution possible when she discovered she was pregnant again four years after Caroline's birth. At thirty-five she was considered a high risk pregnancy, even more so in light of Caroline's condition. Yet Jim and Karrie were very excited about the new baby. "I just want her to come out pink and healthy and wonderfully typical," Karrie said.

An ultrasound at twenty-five weeks brought their dreams crashing down. "I'm so sorry," the doctors informed them, "but the brain has stopped growing. What would you like to do?"

"Excuse me?" Jim asked.

"Regarding the pregnancy and the condition of the fetus," the doctor continued.

Jim and Karrie knew what he was suggesting. Right after Caroline's diagnosis, Karrie had scoured the internet, looking for all the information she could find regarding her daughter's condition. Officially, it is known as microcephaly, which literally means small head. Most of the sites and blogs she came across recommended abortion when the condition was found in utero. That's why Karrie stopped reading sites and blogs about microcephaly long ago. Instead of getting caught up in the experiences of others, she and Jim both made up their minds to take it one day at a time with the faith that they could provide the love and care their daughter needs. Now both were rocked by the news that the healthy baby girl they prayed for was not to be. However, that news did not change their resolve.

"Nothing has changed. She's still our baby girl. Now we know what we're dealing with after our daughter is born," Jim replied.

As firm as they sounded in the doctor's office, they still battled severe grief immediately after receiving the diagnosis. Every family in their position does. All of the hopes and dreams parents naturally have when they discover a child is on its way are snatched away from them the moment the doctor delivers the bad news. Many parents never recover. Jim and Karrie had made peace with Caroline's condition. They grieved the loss of their dreams for their daughter and battled through the questions of "why" and "how" and "what now." Then they stopped grieving and embraced the life they'd been given. Like every parent must, they adjusted their expectations and loved and accepted their daughter for who she was rather than grieving who she was not nor ever would be.

But how does anyone work through the process a second time? Both so wanted a healthy child, even more so because of Caroline's condition. Now they found themselves right back to where they'd been when the neurologist delivered Caroline's crushing diagnosis.

In the midst of their grief and wondering why they had to endure such pain a second time, their eight year old daughter, Kat, walked into the room. She knew her mom and dad were sad. Placing her arm on her mother's shoulder, Kat looked at her with all the sincerity an eight year old can muster and said, "Mom, maybe we did such a good job with Caroline that God gave us another one."

That was all Jim and Karrie needed to pull them out of their grief and set their sights on walking through the known unknown that lay before them.

However, raising two special needs children with severe disabilities does not double the work of raising one special needs child with a severe disability. No, it multiplies it by a factor of at least four. Although Anna and Caroline shared the same condition, their severity differed a great deal. Where Caroline had escaped the most severe complications of microcephaly, Anna was not so fortunate. Early on she cooed and kicked and seemed happy, but it did not last. For the next five years, whatever could go wrong, did go wrong.

Jim and Karrie worked to take it all in stride. Right after Caroline's diagnosis, they made up their minds that their family would not be defined by their special needs children. Not long after Anna came along, they took the entire family on a trip to Florida from their home in Arizona by way of New Orleans. They loaded their four children into the plane along with all of Caroline and Anna's special equipment, including food, pumps, orthotics, and all the other equipment that was simply business as usual in their home. The family looked like a moving crew dragging all their equipment through the airports. Halfway through the trip Jim and Karrie made up their minds to never do this to their children again. No one was able to fully enjoy the trip, especially not Caroline nor Anna.

As Anna grew older, her condition deteriorated. She especially suffered from pulmonary and orthopedic problems. The two conditions conspired against Anna, resulting in regular trips to the hospital for surgeries and procedures. At the age of five her rib cage essentially collapsed in on her lungs, making it nearly impossible for her to breathe. Once again they found themselves in a specialist's office. Unlike the doctor who delivered Caroline's diagnosis, this surgeon refused to let Anna's condition deter him. He saw the family's distress and vowed to do whatever he could to save her. "Her rib cage refuses to let her lungs expand," he explained. "However, we can go in and give her a new, titanium rib cage that will expand and let her breath like normal."

"H...h...how?" Jim stammered.

"We will remove her existing rib cage and a portion of her spine and replace them. It is a very complicated procedure, but it is possible. The entire operation will take about sixteen hours."

Karrie looked down at her little girl. With all of her struggles through her five years of life, Anna was much smaller than a typical five year old. She only weighed twenty pounds, and seemed even more fragile than her size. Karrie looked up at Jim, tears welling up in her eyes. "Let my wife and I talk it over," Jim said.

After the surgeon left the room, Karrie said, "I can't do that to Anna. Putting her through so much just seems inhuman."

Jim reached down and stroked Anna's hair. "I, uh," he could hardly get the words out, "I agree," he said.

"She can't survive sixteen hours on an operating table. I do not want her dying in such a cold place with no one she knows near her, filled with sounds she doesn't recognize. Let's take her home, Jim. Let's take our little angel home."

Jim felt an odd combination of intense grief and relief. A voice in the back of his brain tried to make him feel guilty, as if he was giving up when he should keep on fighting, but he did not give in to it. He knew he was not giving up. Instead, he felt an overwhelming peace that came from accepting the inevitable. "Home is where she needs to be. I'll tell the doctors our decision," he said.

When they arrived home, they tucked Anna into her bed next to her sister. Joe crawled onto the bed and wrapped his arms around his little sister. Over the next three days, Jim, Karrie, Kat and Joe took turns holding Anna. They sang to her and talked to her and loved her as her life slowly slipped away. Every hour they gave her the medicines the hospital had prescribed to minimize her pain. It was all they could do. When they knew the end was at hand, each one whispered their goodbyes. Karrie took Anna in her arms and held her close as Anna's heart finally gave out, a moment both tragic and beautiful.

Not long after Anna's death, a friend came to Karrie and said, "I have a project I would love for you to get involved in." Karrie already served on the board of one charity in the Phoenix area, but she did not feel like she had time for another. Yet, she knew she needed to stay busy as she dealt with the overwhelming grief of Anna's death.

"I don't know," Karrie said. "A lot of days it takes everything in me just to get out of bed. After Anna..." her voice trailed off.

"Just come with me to a community breakfast Saturday morning. No commitment. You aren't signing up for anything. Just come and hear what they are about," the friend said.

Karrie was hesitant, but said yes. "What is this project called, any-way?" she asked.

"Ryan House," the friend replied.

On the morning of the breakfast, Karrie listened as Jonathan Cottor shared his family's story. He talked about Ryan's diagnosis and the way it changed his family's life. Karrie could relate all too well. Then he talked about Helen House in England and the difference it had made. As he talked about Helen House, and the services it offered, Karrie wished a place like that had been available for her family through Anna's ordeal. Then Jonathan shared his vision for building a similar house, Ryan House, in downtown Phoenix. "My wife, Holly, and I have been working to make this dream a reality for six years now, and our board of directors has been in place for five. Construction has started and we plan to be open next year," he said.

By the time the breakfast was over Karrie was hooked. When she told Jim about Ryan House, he was hooked as well. Within a matter of months, both became members of the board of directors. They brought a unique perspective to a board made up of community leaders and movers and shakers. Outside of the Cottors, they were the only members of the board with firsthand experience of raising a child with a life threatening condition. And they were the only members of the board who had had to say goodbye to a child with the type of condition for which Ryan House was being built.

But that wasn't the only appeal of getting involved with Ryan House. Jim and Karrie had an advantage over many families like theirs. From the moment they received Caroline's diagnosis, a community of family and friends surrounded them and helped in any way they could. When Anna was two and Caroline six, one of Jim's business partners threw a party for the family that turned into a fundraiser attended by nearly three hundred people. They were then able to buy a handicap equipped van as well as hire nursing care to come into the home for short periods to take care of Anna and Caroline. That enabled Jim and Karrie to go to all their oldest children's ball games and recitals. Unfortunately, many families who receive an unexpected diagnosis do not have a strong support network. Conditions like microcephaly do not discriminate. They strike rich, poor and middle class; strong marriages and couples tottering on the edge of divorce as well as single parent households.

Because conditions like microcephaly do not discriminate, neither does Ryan House. Its services are offered at no charge to any and every family with a child with a life threatening condition. At the time Jim and Karrie joined the board, the construction of the home was financed completely through donations and grants but that is only part of the story. All of the day to day operations of the House are also financed through donations and community support. Insurance plans do not cover the services Ryan House offers. That is why Jim and Karrie wanted to become active members of the board of directors. They wanted to do more than offer the unique perspective of parents with a special needs child. As soon as they joined the board, they got involved in helping raise money to both build and sustain the vision of Ryan House.

When Ryan House finally opened, Caroline was one of the first guests. Her first solo stay was much harder on Jim and Karrie than it was on Caroline. While Caroline enjoyed the hydrotherapy pool and the music therapy, Karrie spent her time worrying about her little girl. Over the course of a two night stay, Karrie called Ryan House over ten times. Each time she heard the same reassuring words, "Caroline is fine. She's in the sensory room with one of our volunteers listening to music. Would you like to talk to the volunteer?"

"No. That's okay. I just needed to check on her." Karrie replied.

"Call any time," came the reply.

An hour or two later Karrie called again and had basically the same conversation once more. She tried to focus on her time with Jim, Kat and Joe, but it was hard for her to relax and trust someone else to care for Caroline. Even so, she knew the family needed a break. Once they returned to Ryan House to pick up Caroline, they understood that Caroline needed a break from them as well. She was exhausted, but very, very happy.

While Jim and Karrie loaded up Caroline's things, Joe walked around checking out all the rooms. When he returned to her room he said, "Wow, Caroline, you're lucky. I wish I could stay here." It was a very normal, honest conversation that siblings have with one another. Yet it touched Jim and Karrie deeply for it was the first time either of their older children had had this conversation with their little sister. In that moment Ryan House ceased being a House. For Jim and Karrie and Caroline, it was Home.

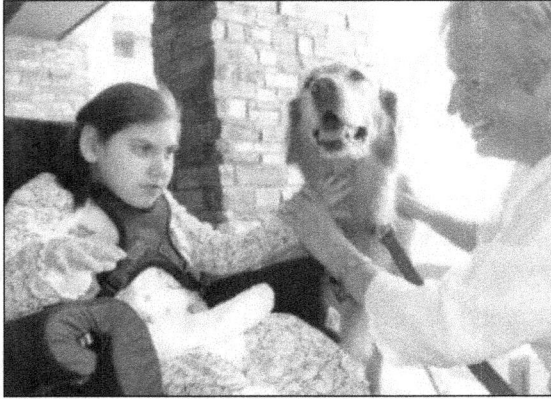

Caroline Pierson enjoying time with Pet Connections volunteer Jan Newman and a furry friend, Hena

Chapter Three

"Wouldn't it be nice..."

THE MOMENT HOLLY'S CELL RANG, she knew what had happened. She stood and moved closer to the train door. *I knew I should have stayed home* she said to herself as she pressed the green send button. "What's wrong?" she said.

"I'm in the ER with Ryan," Jonathan said. "It looks like they're going to admit him."

"I'll get off at the next station and head that way."

"Okay. I'll see you when you get here"."

"Yeah. Okay." Holly hung up and dropped her phone in her purse. "Why did I leave him?!" she yelled at herself.

Ryan had come down with a cold a few days earlier. The cold caused a fever, but it responded to Calpol (the UK equivalent of Tylenol). Even though the fever spiked earlier in the day, the Calpol soon brought it down to a manageable level. Holly saw no reason to cancel her plans. Months earlier she bought tickets to the musical "Mama Mia" for herself and an aunt and cousin from Germany. When Ryan's fever dropped Jonathan reassured her he would take good care of Ryan. Holly had no doubts that he would. Now she kicked herself for treating Ryan's cold like one of Ethan's. *He's too weak to fight these things off. I have to be more proactive.*

Her trip to the hospital took just over half an hour, yet to Holly it seemed much longer. Sitting on a train alone, her mind kept going back to their conversation with the doctor at Helen House less than a week before. *"You will observe changes over time that will give you a sense that he's getting weaker and death may be nearing,"* the doctor had said. Holly couldn't help but think this may have been exactly what he was talking about.

At the hospital, she found Jonathan who filled her in on what he knew. "His chest x-ray shows the lower left lobe of his lung has collapsed."

"Oh my God," she said. "Can they open it back up?"

"They don't know," Jonathan said. "They started IV antibiotics to treat his pneumonia. Now all we can do is wait."

"Do you think...?" Holly couldn't finish the sentence, but Jonathan knew what she was asking.

"I don't know. I don't want to let my mind go there." But it had. Jonathan had already started preparing himself for the news that this was the beginning of the end.

But this was not the beginning of the end. Ryan immediately responded to the antibiotics and was released the next day. Another bout with pneumonia followed a few months later, and another not long after that. With each trip to the ER, Jonathan and Holly braced themselves for the worst, then celebrated when he bounced back. After a while, their minds stopped running to the worst case scenario and they started expecting him to recover. And he always did.

However, the continuing cycle of health scares just confirmed a decision the two of them already felt pushed to make: They needed to move back to the States sooner rather than later. Ryan's health was only part of the equation. Jonathan's job situation had deteriorated. The company that moved the Cottors to London had been absorbed by a larger corporation. As a result of the merger, his previous job responsibilities disappeared. He was reassigned but the handwriting was on the wall. The only way to stay with the company and keep doing what he had always done was to move to Geneva, Switzerland, as part of a purely European team. Accepting the job in Geneva meant becoming a European immigrant rather than an American expatriate living temporarily abroad. He had the option of moving back to the company's home office in Minneapolis, which was where they lived before the move to London. However, relocating to Minneapolis meant he would be immediately laid off. Jonathan started sending out resumés instead.

Prolonged job uncertainty combined with Ryan's illness made Jonathan and Holly feel like their world had crashed around them. They knew they could not survive on their own. Every trip to the ER reminded them of how they needed the kind of support only family can give. On top of that, neither Holly nor Jonathan could stand the thought of depriving the grandparents and aunts, uncles, and cousins the privilege of spending as much time with

Ryan as they possibly could. They felt their only option was to move back to Arizona, surround themselves with family, and love their sons as they tried to live as normally as possible under very abnormal circumstances.

The latter extended a decision they made right after Ryan's diagnosis – life did not stop with the words Spinal Muscular Atrophy. The Cottors were determined not to live their lives like they were attending a funeral that had not yet happened. While living in London they took family trips to Paris and Italy and all the other places they knew they might never get to see again. They approached their prospective move to Phoenix in the same way. They were not moving there to wait for Ryan to die. No, they were going back to Arizona to live. But first, Jonathan had to find a job and the family had to find a place to live.

Just over a month after Ryan's first major bout with pneumonia, the family flew to Arizona for a combination Christmas/job search/home shopping trip. Every time they returned to the Phoenix area, all their extended family did their best to come see them, along with all the family's lifelong friends. Sharon focused on the Phoenix area, while Holly's parents, Judi and Budd Busche, saw to it that Tucson friends and family had their share of time, too. Each grandparent worked the phones and arranged get-togethers to make sure everyone important to the family saw Ryan. The reunions always had a greater sense of urgency than simply getting together with family after a prolonged absence. No one knew whether this might be the last time they would get to see Ryan. The oxygen tank that accompanied Ryan on the plane because of his recent bout with pneumonia only increased the air of uncertainty.

About halfway through the Cottors' Christmas visit, Diane Eckstein dropped by Bob and Sharon's house. Diane and her husband John were long-time friends of the Cottors. After a few minutes of small talk, Diane asked Holly, "How are you and Jonathan doing *really* with everything that is going on? You have your hands full with Ethan, and now Ryan's diagnosis..."

"Well, you know, we just sort of do what we have to do," Holly said, not really answering the question.

"We both know there's more to it than that," Diane replied.

Holly laughed. "You're right. Honestly, I'm not really sure how we've kept it together. This has been a roller coaster ride with very few highs and way too many lows. We braced ourselves for the end with his pneumonia and collapsed lung last month, but then he surprised us and bounced out of the hospital the next day. His muscles may be weak because of SMA but he's a very strong little boy."

Diane nodded her head, watching Ryan. "I cannot imagine."

"We found a place, though, that's been a godsend. There's a children's hospice in Oxford called Helen House where we've gone for respite. Ryan really seems to like it, and Jonathan and I love it. I think Ethan feels like he's found another Disneyland with the special features and things he can play with!"

The word "hospice" piqued Diane's interest. Her father-in-law had been the first medical director for Hospice of the Valley, the largest not-for-profit hospice organization in Arizona and one of the largest in the country. "That doesn't sound like the typical American hospice," she said.

"It's set up for kids with prognoses like Ryan's, not just for end-of-life care," Holly said. "But you know, the thing that is so great about Helen House is that when we're there, we're normal. Every family there is dealing with the same kind of issues we deal with, a lot of them a lot worse than us. There's just a feeling there that I can hardly describe. All the families, we're just sort of in this thing together. There it's not odd to have a special needs child or a child in a wheelchair or to have a discussion about the death of a child. I don't know how we could survive without it. I'm really going to miss it when we move back here. It would be nice if we had something like it in Phoenix."

"Why can't we?" Diane asked.

"I don't know. I wish we could," Holly replied.

"This really sounds like something I'd like you to share with the Executive Director of Hospice of the Valley, Susan Levine, when you move back. Why don't you take some time getting settled when you return and, if you'd like to meet with her, let me know. I'll do whatever I can to help make it happen," Diane said.

Holly didn't think too much about the conversation with Diane after they returned to London. They had too much to do. Jonathan accepted a job in Phoenix and the two of them got ready for the move. They stayed at Helen House one last time as a family, then had Ryan stay there on his own while they finished packing for the move. Leaving Ryan by himself marked a turning point for the Cottors. He was approaching his second birthday, something the doctors warned them he would probably never see. Yet, every day he seemed to be growing stronger, not weaker. Even with the frequent trips to the ER, nothing about his condition made them think the end was at hand. Leaving Ryan at Helen House alone showed both the level of trust the Cottors had developed with the staff there and also a step back, however small, from the brink where they felt certain they could lose their son at any moment.

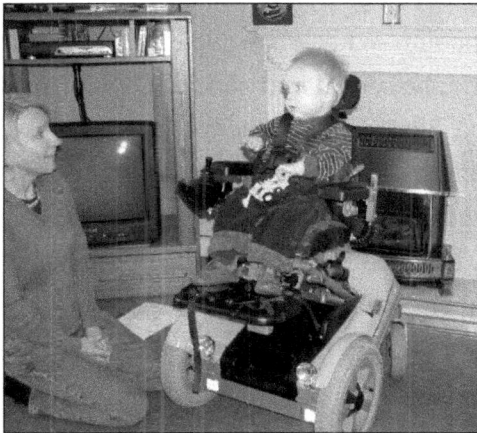

Ryan's first moment in a wheelchair

Two days before leaving the UK for good, the Cottors took another step toward normalcy. At an age when most children Ryan's age have started walking, he, too, became mobile. Jonathan and Holly bought him a Permobil Koala pediatric power wheelchair designed specifically for Ryan and his SMA. When they placed him in the chair for the first time, Ryan grabbed the joystick and the chair moved forward. Tears filled their eyes. These were his first "steps". For his first week or so, his chair didn't go forward very often. Most of the time he pulled back on the stick and did backward circles. Before long, however, he got the hang of it and was on his way. From time to time he bumped into walls but not often. Even at such a young age, Ryan and the chair had become one. His world opened up when he became mobile.

The Cottors moved home to Phoenix in March, 2003. One month later they celebrated a milestone they never expected to experience: Ryan turned two. A week before his birthday, Holly asked, "What do you want for breakfast on your birthday?"

"Cake," Ryan replied.

"We'll have cake at your party. What do you want for breakfast in the morning?"

"Cake!"

The two of them had the same conversation every day for a week. When he woke up on the morning of his birthday, he woke up looking for cake. Holly did not disappoint. While she saved the actual birthday cake for the party later in the day, she served him pancakes with frosting for breakfast.

Bob and Sharon hosted the birthday party. A Bob the Builder Happy Birthday banner hung on a wall while the dining room table had a Bob the Builder Happy Birthday table cloth over it upon which sat a Bob the Builder birthday cake. They also had Bob the Builder cups and hats and anything else Bob the Builder birthday-related they could find. Family and friends filled the house. Cousins near Ryan and Ethan's ages ran around laughing and playing, with Ryan doing his best to keep up in his Koala.

As the party scene unfolded, Jonathan stood back and took a deep breath. *Eighty percent of children with the most severe form of SMA do not survive to their second birthday*, echoed in his head. *Eighty percent don't, but Ryan did!* Ethan darted past him, with Ryan on his heels. He still had trouble making the chair go where he wanted it to go, but he had such a look of determination on his face that it was clear he was going to conquer this thing. Watching the scene unfold, a wave of emotion swept over Jonathan. Never in his wildest dreams did he ever think he would watch his boys chasing one another through the house like typical brothers do. He looked across the room at Holly. She was busy filling Bob the Builder cups with soda. She happened to look up and notice Jonathan staring at her. When their eyes met, he mouthed, "He did it."

She smiled back, both of them struggling to hold themselves together.

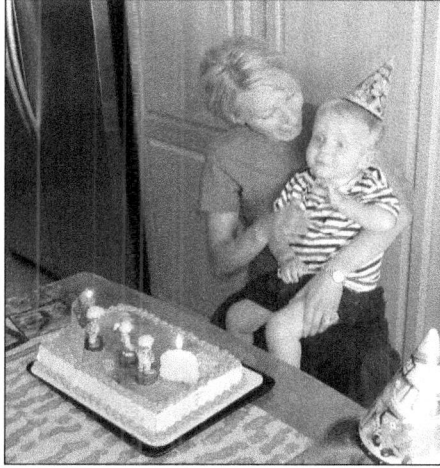

Ryan turns 2!

Their first few months in Arizona felt like a prolonged moving period. They lived temporarily in an apartment while looking for a house. Once they found a house, Budd worked with Jonathan to build ramps and other modifications to make their home as wheelchair friendly as possible. Jonathan busied himself settling into his new job while Holly spent much of her time finding the right doctors and treatment facilities for Ryan's condition. There was also the question of how they could afford Ryan's care. Before moving back to Arizona, they'd heard horror stories of how tight medical insurance was in Arizona. Since Ryan had a major pre-existing condition, they feared they would not be able to find a company that would cover them, or, if they did, the premiums would be so expensive they would not be able to afford them. In fact, a friend with a child with special needs had faced $5,000 a month premiums.

Fortunately, they soon discovered Arizona is one of the best states in the nation for families like theirs. The state's Medicaid system supports children with special medical needs. The Cottors did not have to cover the expense of Ryan's care themselves, which made it possible for them to function financially.

Throughout these months, Holly and Jonathan often talked about how they wished they could spend a weekend at Helen House. While family and friends helped all they could, nothing compared to the sense of belonging they felt there. Whenever someone asked them what they missed most about London, the answer was always the same: Helen House.

Once Holly and Jonathan finally moved into their house and were reasonably settled, Sharon called an extended family meeting. Holly's parents, Judi and Budd Busche, were also there. Sharon got the family meeting going. "Something that Bob and I have strongly believed in throughout our lives and professional careers is that 'family comes first.' We want to support you in the ways that can be most helpful to the four of you," she announced. Given her experience as a family therapist, she knew the families that survive a child's prolonged illness are those that tackle the condition as a unified team. The bigger the team, the more successful they are. Divorce rates for couples with children with life threatening conditions hover around ninety percent.

"I think you're doing a pretty good job already," Jonathan answered. "You're all great with the boys, and you're always there to do whatever we need."

"Now that's all well and good but what do you need the most?" Sharon replied.

"You can bring a children's hospice over from London for us," Holly said with a laugh.

"Okay," Bob said, "we'll do it."

"Budd, you've built several homes," Sharon said. "You ought to just build one here," she said jokingly.

"I guess it's not out of the question," Budd exclaimed.

"I was thinking Budd's next house would be his final, but THIS house sounds like it would be a dream house for many. Our final house can wait!" Judi added.

Holly jumped in. "I don't think our family building a hospice is really an option. Although I would love to have one here, there's a lot more to it than just putting up a building."

"We don't have to build it," Sharon replied, "but maybe someone will."

Holly smiled. "Maybe," she said, letting the conversation die there. "Now back to what you guys can do to help us."

Later that evening, after Holly and Jonathan had returned home, Holly turned to Jonathan and said, "I'm going to call Diane Eckstein tomorrow."

"Really?" Jonathan replied.

"I think it's time."

"I think that's a good idea," Jonathan said.

"She is very connected to Hospice of the Valley. They do pediatric hospice already. Maybe they would be interested in expanding the definition of what they do for kids."

"It's a place to start," Jonathan said.

"Then let's see what happens," Holly said. "You never know."

"No, you never know," Jonathan said.

Chapter Four

"I think we should go for it."

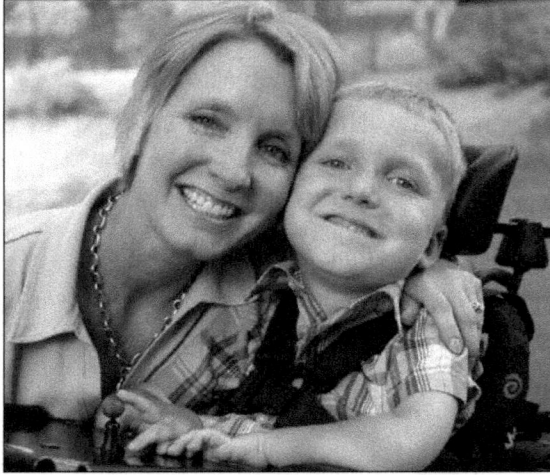

Holly and Ryan

"SHALL I TAKE YOU TO Mrs. Levine's table?" the waiter asked. "I believe she is expecting you, correct?"

"Yes she is. Thank you," Diane Eckstein replied.

"Follow me, please," the waiter said.

"Certainly," Diane said. She looked over at Holly. "There's no need to be nervous. You're going to love Susan."

"That's easy for you to say," Holly said. "I can't believe we are doing this."

Diane laughed. "You'll be fine. Don't worry. Just explain everything to her the way you did for me. You convinced me, didn't you?"

Holly let out a sigh. "I guess so."

They followed the waiter through the maze of tables in Bistro 24, the in-house restaurant at the Ritz Carlton Hotel in Phoenix. Holly's legs felt heavy. She could hear her heart beating in her ears. No matter how many times she told herself not to be nervous, she could not calm herself. In Phoenix, meeting Susan Levine, her lunch appointment for today, was like meeting royalty. Not only had Susan established herself as one of the most influential women in the community through her leadership of Hospice of the Valley, the largest single site hospice organization in the nation, she also carried a mystique as Barry Goldwater's widow. The recipient of many local and national awards, the Arizona Centennial Legacy Project later named her one of Arizona's forty-eight most intriguing women. (Forty-eight because Arizona was the forty-eighth state.)

Diane had no qualms about setting up this meeting between Holly and Susan. She'd known Susan for a very long time and had crossed paths with her on several other projects.

"Here you are, ladies," the waiter said as they reached Susan's table. "Your server will be with you in just a moment."

"Thank you," Diane said. Then motioning toward Holly, she said, "Susan, this is Holly Cottor."

Susan stood and reached across the table to shake Holly's hand. For a split second, Holly considered grabbing a napkin and wiping away the sweat from her own palm before taking Susan's hand, but thought better of it. "So glad to meet you," Susan said. "Please, have a seat. Diane told me you've had a very moving experience with a children's hospice. Why don't you tell me about it."

After taking a deep breath to calm her nerves, Holly proceeded to tell Susan her story of Ryan's diagnosis while they lived in England and what it was like over the first several months trying to care for him while living with the fear of his death. Then she began talking about Helen House and the impact it made on their family. As she described Helen House, she passed over photos she'd found online of the different rooms, including the bedrooms and specialty rooms. She also handed Susan one of the flyers the staff at Helen House gave her when she toured the house the first time.

The more Holly talked, the more at ease she grew. Their server came and took their order. Holly paused just long enough to order a salad, and then dove back into her presentation. Susan stopped her several times to ask questions while she looked over the materials Holly brought along. The food arrived, but Holly did not feel like eating. She finished her presentation by saying, "There are no children's hospices that provide palliative care here in the states but I believe that needs to change. I know there are a lot of families just like ours out there for whom a place like this would be a godsend."

"You're probably right," Susan said. "This is all very impressive. So what would you like from me?"

Holly glanced over at Diane, unsure of what to say. Diane spoke up. "Hospice of the Valley has offered children's hospice for a long time. I thought you may be able to give us some advice about where to start in trying to build a children's hospice that would provide respite care to families in Phoenix."

Susan nodded her head. "Let me give that a little thought. Do you want to know how to start this yourself or how to get someone else interested in building it?"

"I just want to see it happen whatever it takes," Holly said. "I, obviously, am not equipped to go out and start something of this size. I think it would be best for an established organization to take the lead. I don't see any other way to make it happen."

"You might be surprised," Susan said with a smile. "Now, as for Hospice of the Valley, this is not something I think we would be interested in doing right now. But that doesn't mean I don't think it is a good idea. Have you already looked around to see what programs are out there?"

Holly shook her head. "No, not yet."

"I think that would be the place to start. In fact, after we finish here why don't we go over to HOV's Coronado Home? You can meet a boy who is receiving hospice care there." Susan said. "After that, you are more than welcome to come by our office and get a feel for how we do things. You're talking about starting a hospice, which is what we do."

"I don't know about calling it a hospice. Do you think people are ready for the idea of a hospice for children?" Holly asked.

"I think you should call it what it is," Susan replied. "Don't you?"

"I'm not sure. I am afraid most people will think it sounds like throwing in the towel and waiting for a child to die."

Susan smiled. "You need to see how we do hospice. It's not what you think," Susan said.

Holly and Diane spent the rest of the afternoon touring HOV's Coronado Home and peppering Susan with questions. While Coronado Home was beautiful, it did not have the look and feel of Helen House. Nor was it set up to provide respite care for tired families struggling with the demands of caring for a special needs child over the long term. As nice as the facility was, it wasn't what Holly was hoping to find. While Coronado Home was equipped to handle children, it wasn't designed *for* them. To Holly, that difference was critical. It was what made Helen House special. Children aren't part of its mission. They *are* its mission.

While at Coronado Home, Holly sat and visited with one school age boy who was dying. Talking to him was very difficult for her. Clearly, the hospice workers had worked hard to personalize his space and make his room something special just for him. A local wish granting organization granted his wish for a stereo system in a very big way. The system took up an entire wall, with speakers that were nearly as tall as the boy. A smile broke out on his face when he pointed over to the stereo. "I like to play it really loud," he grinned.

"It looks like it can shake the walls," Holly said.

"Oh yeah," the boy replied.

After a few minutes, Holly walked out of his room and into the hallway. "Wow, what a brave little boy," she said to Diane who had not gone inside the room. As she said this, she glanced into the room directly across the hall. A very elderly woman lay in the bed. Holly guessed she was probably in her nineties. *I wonder how she likes the stereo?* she asked herself.

Diane noticed Holly staring into the woman's room. "What's wrong?"

"I don't want to be negative because this place is so nice and the workers obviously have gone above and beyond for this little boy but it's just not the same as Helen House. I envision a place where children aren't just welcomed. They need a place where they can be kids without disturbing anyone."

Susan rejoined Holly and Diane and led them to the door. "Well, ladies, what did you think?" she asked.

"The home is beautiful," Holly said, "but..."

"But it's not what you have in mind, correct?" Susan said.

"I'm sorry. I don't mean to be critical."

"No need to apologize," Susan said with a smile. "I understand completely."

"It's just..." Holly paused. Her emotions started to get the best of her. "I'm sure a children's hospice house won't happen here during Ryan's lifetime, but I still think it needs to be built. I know that many other families would be grateful for that type of care."

"I'm sure that it will happen during his lifetime," Susan said.

"That's very nice of you to say," Holly said.

"I'm not just being nice. Let's stay in touch. Feel free to come by our office and take a look around. You can even use our facilities as you explore what's out there."

"I may take you up on your offer," Holly said.

"Please do."

On the drive home after leaving Susan, Holly stared out the passenger window, silent. "Well, what did you think of Susan?" Diane asked.

"She's great," Holly said. "But..."

"But you would have liked for her to have been a little more enthusiastic about the idea, right?"

"Well..."

"Susan is a very good business woman and a strong leader. She's not just going to jump into anything. But she did offer to help any way she could and she made HOV's offices available for you to use."

Holly let out a long sigh. "That's a start. I just...I don't know. There are lots of children's hospices in England. You see them in every community. The culture there, it's so different. People seem to accept the fact that death is part of life, even for children. And they seem to have a better grasp on the fact that doctors can't fix everything. I don't know how anyone can recreate that culture and get people to see the need for a children's hospice right here, in Phoenix."

"Change takes time. Don't get discouraged. I have more people we can talk to. Let me make a couple of calls. Like I told you last year, I will do whatever you need me to do to help make this dream happen. We've hardly even started."

Diane did not share Holly's hesitations. She knew from experience what it took to start from scratch, a service for a need no one else seemed to notice. A social worker by profession, she spent most of her professional life working with children in foster care and with special needs adoptive families. After she and her husband returned to the Phoenix area in the early eighties, she discovered these families did not have the resources available to them that they needed to deal with the unique issues they faced on a daily basis. After receiving more training in family therapy, she and a colleague started their own agency to meet that need. That was part of the reason why she felt so drawn to Holly and the idea of launching a children's hospice in Phoenix. Both special needs adoptive families and families with children with life limiting conditions suffer from high rates of burn out and divorce. After dedicating so much of her life to the former, it just felt natural to do whatever she could to help the latter.

Over the next several weeks Holly spent every spare moment Googling "children's hospice" and "children's palliative care" and "respite for families of children with life limiting conditions." She learned many groups across the United States had attempted to recreate the Helen House model but all had failed. All, that is, but one. To her surprise, she came across a house slated to open early the next year – named George Mark Children's House, after the founder's brothers who each died early, one at sixteen and the other at thirty. The home was located in the Oakland, California area. Holly immediately contacted George Mark Children's House to learn more about how they had succeeded where so many others had failed. The answer was less than encouraging. A single donor had given a huge, multi-million dollar gift both to build and operate the house. Short of finding a wealthy benefactor to bankroll a

Phoenix house, Holly didn't see how their approach to getting the house built could help make one a reality in Arizona. However, she was intrigued to learn how the George Mark team had created an environment open to hospice and palliative care as more than a last resort. The George Mark team invited her to come to California to take a look around, an invitation she planned to accept.

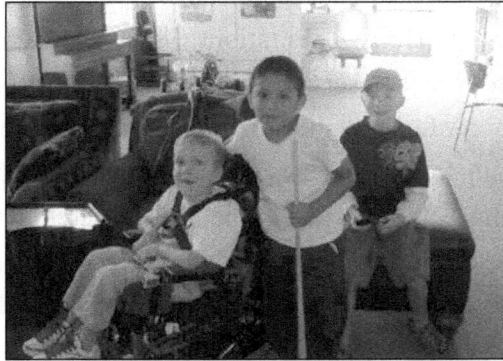

Ryan and his brother, Ethan, with a friend at George Mark Children's House (The Cottor family was able to visit and stay a few days after moving back to AZ).

She also took advantage of Susan's offer to visit HOV's facilities to take a look around. More than anything, she wanted to see for herself what pediatric hospice care in the States looked like. Her and Jonathan's understanding of the word had already evolved during their stays at Helen House in England. Watching the HOV staff in action, she was very encouraged. As in England, she found people who'd made the courageous decision to accept the fact that their childhood conditions could not be cured and then move on with living. She discovered the care administered through hospice mirrored the description of palliative care the doctor at Helen House explained to her and Jonathan during their first visit. While treatments weren't curative in nature, they were just as essential to help patients have the best quality of life possible during their lifetime. In HOV's facilities, she discovered music therapy and aroma therapy along with pet therapy and a variety of other approaches to connect with patients and give them joy. *They haven't given up hope. This is the very definition of hope!* Holly told herself.

A few weeks after her lunch meeting, Susan Levine invited Holly to come and speak to one of HOV's staff meetings and share her experience with Helen House. Her audience included doctors and nurses as well as social workers. After she spoke, a social worker named Karen approached Holly. "You don't know how much your talk meant to me," Karen said. "I've wanted to do more for children like Ryan for a long time." Karen went on to explain how she'd first become acquainted with palliative care while working in Chicago. After she and her husband moved to Phoenix, she went to work at Hospice of the Valley as part of their pediatric hospice team that cared for children in their homes. Spending time with these children brought her face to face with the extreme emotional, physical and spiritual fatigue the families face. That's why the idea of a home that offered respite care so resonated with her.

"I'm going up to San Leandro in a couple of weeks to tour George Mark. Why don't you go with me?" Holly said.

"Let me check my schedule, but I would love to," Karen replied.

Two weeks later, Holly and Karen walked through the doors of the still unfinished George Mark House. "Wow," Holly said, "this looks like a bigger and newer Helen House."

"Really?" Karen said.

"Eight bedrooms that look out on a garden, the family rooms, they definitely followed Helen House's model. Oh, and look at this!" she said as they came to a room on the opposite side of one of the bedrooms. "They included a sensory room like at Helen House. Ryan loved this room when he stayed there."

They walked through the rest of the house, stepping around paint drop cloths and avoiding construction workers putting the finishing touches on the rooms. The kitchen had the same open, inviting set-up that made conversations so easy at Helen House, as did the main living room. However, she was more than a little disappointed when they walked outside to the playground. "The play structure is not wheelchair accessible," she said. "Ethan would be able to enjoy it, but not Ryan."

After their tour, the house director invited Holly and Karen to go out to dinner with some of the staff members and others who, like Holly, were there because they were interested in building children's hospices in their communities. At dinner, Holly found herself seated next to a physician who asked how Holly became interested in George Mark Children's House.

"I have a son with SMA," she told him. "We actually lived in London when he was diagnosed."

"Then you must be familiar with Helen House," he replied.

"Oh yes. We stayed there a few times before we moved back to the States."

"I've not met many people who have stayed there with their children," he said. "Since you've been there, you must have read the book *A House Called Helen*?"

"There's a book?" Holly said.

"A very good book. We couldn't have done what we did here without it," he said. "It tells step by step how they built Helen House. It was the first children's hospice over there, you know. I'm surprised you aren't familiar with the book."

Holly pulled a piece of paper and a pen out of her purse. She wrote the title down. "I'm going to order it as soon as I get back to Phoenix," she said.

When the book arrived in the mail, she devoured it. With each page, a light started to come on. When she first called Diane Eckstein and went with her to meet with Susan Levine, Holly had no thought of actually trying to build a children's hospice herself. The idea seemed impossible. Something so big was more than one family could possibly tackle by themselves. Yet, that was exactly how Helen House started. One tireless nurse, Sister Frances Dominica, uplifted young Helen and her family, extending friendship by offering to care for their child for a short break. That one act of friendship started the process that ultimately resulted not only in Helen House but in children's hospices across England. Actually building the house took a huge community effort but every movement has to start somewhere.

Why not us? Holly asked herself. *Helen House started by offering friendship and care. We are simply looking to do the same. There must be others like Sister Frances in Phoenix.*

Before she even finished reading the book, she told Jonathan, "You have got to read this."

As Jonathan read the book, he became even more excited than Holly. "We can do this," he said to her.

"You know, I think so, too," Holly replied.

"We have to at least try. Let's go for it."

"Okay," Holly said. A wave of emotion swept over her. She felt like bursting out in tears and jumping up and down with excitement all at the same time. "Let's do it," she said.

Even after reading "A House Called Helen" which gave a blueprint for how Helen House came to be, Holly and Jonathan had no way of knowing exactly what lay ahead of them. "Going for it" meant tackling several challenges, the size of which they could not fully appreciate for some time to come.

They knew their first challenge would be money. Neither had any illusion that a project of this size and scope could be pulled off on the cheap. Holly and Jonathan knew that this "House" was no ordinary house. The building had to be equipped to care for very sick children without looking like a house equipped to care for very sick children.

As far as the House itself, the Cottors saw no need to tinker with a model that worked so well across the UK. The House should have eight bedrooms for children, each of which needed to look out on a garden of some sort. The home also needed family suites, perhaps as many as four. The family suites were perhaps the Cottors' favorite part of their experience at Helen House. Staying in the house gave them the opportunity to connect with other families in a way not possible anywhere else. While staying in the home, everyone there felt like family. Anything they built in Phoenix had to create the same atmosphere, which meant building family suites that felt like a real retreat.

The House also needed a large, inviting kitchen and dining area where families could prepare meals and eat together. Like any good home, the House needed a large living room as well as a place for children to go outside and play. Since most of the children have physical restrictions, the playground needed to be fully wheel chair accessible. The home should also include a hydrotherapy room with a large, inviting pool, along with an art room, music room, and a sensory room, all for the children. In addition, they wanted to offer a sanctuary room where families could find a quiet place to deal with the unique challenges which they faced on a daily basis, along with offering a place where they could go as they faced the death of their children. The sanctuary could also double as a chapel for families who wanted to hold their children's memorial services at a place that meant so much to them.

In terms of care, the House needed a central area for the care team that didn't look like a clinical "nurses' station." Working with very ill children required a place where care could be coordinated and meds could be securely stored. The House also needed a spacious bathroom where children with a variety of physical limitations could be bathed and cared for.

On top of all of this, before the first brick could be laid, the house needed a location, preferably near the city center where families could have easy access to restaurants, shows, and other things that would make staying in the home a real vacation. Such a location within a major city would obviously be prime real estate, which meant it would be expensive.

Altogether, they imagined building a House in Phoenix that would carry a price tag in the millions of dollars, all for a place that could only serve eight children and their families at any one time. People and communities often come together to tackle "big" projects. The Cottors wondered if their community would come together for something so important and yet so small in terms of the number of families who would actually use it? Yet the larger impact on the community would be huge.

As large as the price tag seemed, Jonathan and Holly already had an inkling that money would prove to be the smallest obstacle. Far larger would be the challenge of opening people's eyes and minds to the need for the house. First on that list of those to be convinced were the families for whom the home was to be built. Although the word "hospice" no longer carried negative implications for the Cottors, it still did for most people, even those with children with life limiting conditions. Even without using the word "hospice" and instead focusing on respite care, most of these families did not automatically see it as something they needed. Jonathan and Holly understood this all too well. They resisted going to Helen House because they felt they should be able to manage the challenges of Ryan's care on their own. Even after they fell in love with Helen House, they always felt a little guilty about the luxury of rest they received there. They got over their guilt rather quickly, but they knew these same initial feelings would present an obstacle to getting other families like theirs to buy into the concept.

In addition to the challenge of getting families to accept the need for a children's hospice in Phoenix, the medical community presented even greater difficulty. Physicians did not feel comfortable referring children to hospice, especially early on. While many doctors understood the importance of palliative care, most still had trouble focusing on palliative care alone without working tirelessly to prolong a child's life no matter what it took. Like Holly's initial hesitation, when it came to children, many in the medical community saw hospice as a last resort when all hope was lost.

They were not alone. Most Americans think of hospice and end-of-life care as one and the same. Insurance companies reflect this misconception by only covering six months of hospice care. The British children's hospice model was built on the idea that hospice care be given long term, even over the course of years. It openly accepted the fact that children are stricken with diseases and conditions which cannot be cured. Instead of finding a cure at all costs, the UK model works through palliative care to give these children the best quality of life possible for as long or as short as their lives may last.

Creating awareness of the need for a children's hospice in Phoenix meant working to change a philosophy and understanding of death and dying in regard to children. Jonathan and Holly knew this, but they chose not to focus on the size of such a challenge. Otherwise they may well have given up before they even started. In England, this philosophy already existed. Not on this side of the pond. It seemed antithetical to the "can do, we can lick anything" mindset that most Americans believe is as much a part of who we are as baseball and apple pie.

Hand in hand with the challenge of changing the prevailing perception of hospice care for children, was the challenge of getting the community as a whole to buy into the need to build and sustain a House in Phoenix. In some ways, building the House would be the easy part. People rally to causes. They come together to make something happen. But the real test of the community's buy-in would come years after the House was built, if it were ever built. Would the community value this place so much that it would make sure the doors never closed? The question went back to the challenge of money. Neither Jonathan nor Holly could put a price tag on the annual operating cost for a House like this, but they knew it would be expensive. The only way to keep the House going was to get the community to accept it to such a degree that they would not let it fail. As a marketer, Jonathan had some ideas how to make this happen, but he knew one family could not do this alone.

Finally, they faced the challenge of clearly communicating the vision of the House they hoped to build, while also making sure the vision did not suffer dilution or change through the planning and building process. When asked to describe in one sentence the house they hoped to build, Jonathan gave a simple, two word answer: Helen House. More important than the building layout and design, both he and Holly uncompromisingly wanted to recreate the culture of Helen House. *It had to be a House devoted to providing respite and palliative care to children with life-threatening conditions along with end-of-life care as needed.* They envisioned a place with an atmosphere of openness, collaboration and camaraderie among the affected families.

If the House was to truly be a place of respite for these children, it had to look and feel like a home, not a medical facility. They knew from experience that these families had enough of medical facilities. Anything that smacked of doctors, nurses, needles and treatments would immediately make these children retreat in fear. This House had to do the opposite. The staff, therefore, had to dress casually, not like medical professionals. Although the House had to have some level of medical equipment on site, it could not be visible. Visiting this House had to feel like going to grandma's house.

The House also had to be available to all families who needed it at no charge. Every part of life is incredibly expensive for families with children with life limiting conditions. From medical care to specialized medical equipment to equipping their homes for wheelchairs as well as the need for wheelchair accessible vehicles, everything they needed to function as close to normal as possible comes at a high price. For this House to give a real break, it must alleviate, not add to, the financial worries that were a daily part of these families' lives.

The insistence on making the House available at no charge carried with it the danger that somewhere down the road the House's leadership might be tempted to expand the House's purpose in order to create revenue streams to finance the operation. This was not simply a theoretical danger; it was a challenge every non-profit with a clearly defined, and limited, mission statement faces. It takes money to keep the doors open, and that money must come from somewhere. While insurance companies will pay for end-of-life care, they will not pay for respite care. Based on the experience of the children's hospices in England, the vast majority of the House's use will fall under respite and will therefore not be covered by insurance companies. That means the House will face the ongoing challenge of staying true to its original vision, while also raising the money needed for the day-to-day operation of the House. Jonathan knew this challenge lay not just in the future, but even through the planning and building process. Those who came on board would naturally look ahead to sustainability, which would bring this discussion front and center.

All of these challenges lay ahead as the Cottors decided to go for it. If they had fully understood the breadth of each, they may well have had second thoughts. But that's the beauty of pursuing a vision: You go forward firm, in the conviction that your vision is bigger than any of the obstacles you may face.

Santana

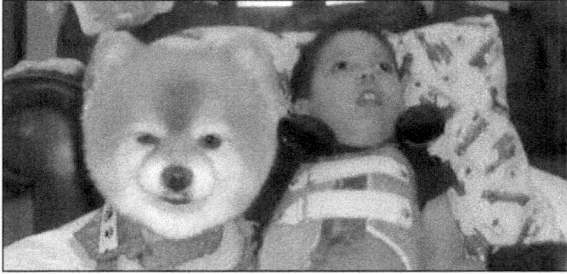

Pet Connections: "Baer" with Santana

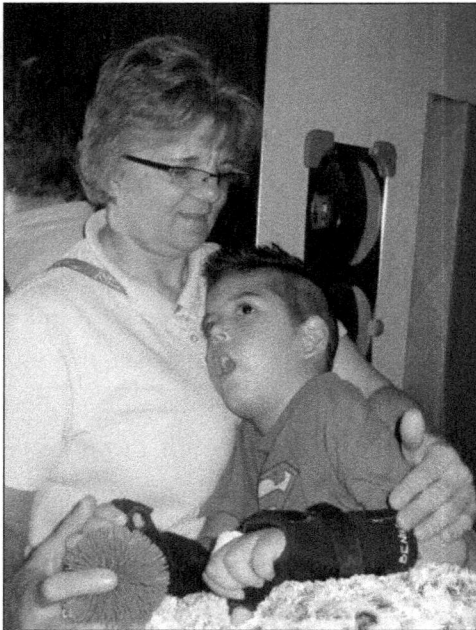

Kasia and Santana enjoying the Sensory Room

Lindsey and James had just sat down to eat when his phone rang. "Hold on a minute she's right here," James said as he passed the phone to his wife. "It's your stepmom. Probably has a question about the boys." Lindsey and James had left their two sons, Jett and Santana, with her father and stepmother for the weekend while they helped some friends move. They were out for brunch before going back to the house and loading their friends' stuff into a truck. Lindsey didn't mind the delay. She wasn't in a big hurry to start carrying boxes.

"Why didn't she call me?" Lindsey asked.

"Who knows," James said, handing her the phone.

"Hey, what's up?" she said. "Wait..." her countenance fell. James stood up and moved toward her. "Slow down. What happened...? How?...Where is he now? ..Okay, we're on our way." She hung up the call and looked up, the blood had washed out of her face.

"What is it?" James asked.

"It's Santana," she said, barely able to get the words out. "There's been an accident."

"What happened?'

"She couldn't tell me. She and my dad were out Christmas shopping and they left the boys with her niece. My brother called my mom from their house and told her there was some sort of accident. He doesn't even know exactly what happened. Apparently my brother was down at the shop when one of the neighbors called asking him why there was yellow police tape around the house."

"He raced up to the house, but by the time he got there the ambulance was gone with Santana in it."

"Which hospital did they take him to?" James asked.

"I guess Phoenix Children's."

"Let's go," James said.

A short time later, Lindsey pounded on the Phoenix Children's Hospital emergency room reception desk. "Santana Black. S-A-N-T-A-N-A B-L-A-C-K! It's not that hard of a name to find. Now let me see my son!"

"I'm sorry, ma'am," the receptionist said, "but I don't have anyone here by that name."

"He has to be here. An ambulance just brought him in."

"Are you sure he's here? They may have taken him to one of the other hospitals in the area. Have you tried the pediatric unit at St. Joe's."

Lindsey started to collapse, but James put his arm around her to hold her up. "We'll try there," he said. "Thank you."

When they arrived at St. Joseph's hospital, they were immediately ushered into a large conference room. "Have a seat and the doctors will be right in," they were told. Lindsey and James sat down at the long table that filled the room. An eternity passed. The room felt very cold and sterile.

Finally, a doctor came in. "Mr. and Mrs. Black, I'm afraid I don't have very good news. Your son, Santana, nearly drowned today. As of yet it is unclear how long he was under the water and deprived of oxygen. I can tell you that he had to be revived at the scene. He was clinically dead for at least thirty minutes." Lindsey started to weep. "The only reason he is still alive is because it's December and the water was very cold."

"Is he, uh," James cleared his throat, "is my son going to make it?"

"Right now I can't tell you which way the coin is going to fall. He is either going to live or die tonight. If he survives tonight, his odds of survival long term improve. But I have to be honest with you. Given what your son has gone through, his chances don't look good right now."

"Can I see my little boy?" Lindsey asked.

"Not yet," the doctor said. "I'm sorry, but we can't have you in there while we're working on him."

"I understand," she said.

Two hours later, Lindsey and James were ushered into the intensive care unit, along with her father and step mother. They slowly approached Santana's bed. Machines whirred around them. Wires hung from all over his body. A tube came up out of his mouth and connected to the respirator which was breathing for him. His chest went up and down almost violently.

The family gathered around his bed. For a moment, they thought they were in the wrong room. Their twenty-two month old toddler did not look like himself. His entire body was bloated and his skin still had a bluish – purplish tint. "Santana, baby," Lindsey said as she stroked his hair. He did not respond. She looked up at her husband who moved over close and took her hand.

"God, I pray you will heal my son," he started to pray. The rest of the family joined in. At this point, prayer was their only hope for his survival. God answered their prayers, but life was never going to be the same for any of them.

Six weeks after the accident, Lindsey and James loaded Santana into their car for the drive home. While they were thrilled their son was alive, this was not the same child they left at Lindsey's father's house on December 15, 2006. Santana had always been an incredibly active child. He and his big brother constantly found ways to get into mischief. One afternoon Lindsey walked into their game room only to find Santana standing in the middle of what looked like a snow storm. Somehow, he and his brother had found a way to dismantle an oversized bean bag chair. "Santana, what happened?" Lindsey said in that panicked mom's voice all mothers use. He flashed a smile that made her heart melt. Her anger turned to laughter. "You are such a little charmer with that smile of yours," she said with a laugh.

Santana lost his smile the day he fell into her father's pool chasing the toy stroller he'd accidentally pushed into the water. Even though the pool had a fence around one side, he'd managed to get to it through a side door out of the garage where he'd been playing with his brother. First responders estimate he was under water for at least twenty minutes. His brain was deprived of oxygen for somewhere between forty-five and fifty minutes. As a result, he suffered a severe brain injury that left him unable to walk or talk or care for himself in any way. He came off the ventilator in less than a week, which was a miracle in itself. Surgeons inserted a G-tube and later performed another procedure after he had trouble holding food down. Lindsey learned to perform the deep suction procedure he needed to clear his lungs, as well as how to monitor his oxygen levels. The brain injury also caused all his muscles to pull up tight, causing his body to try to bend like a backwards C. He required a regimen of medications to relax his body enough for him to be placed in an upright position.

Therefore, bringing Santana home after his six weeks in the hospital was like bringing home a newborn. Fitting him into his car seat was a challenge as his contracted muscles fought against settling into a seated position. His blood pressure spiked and phlegm had to be suctioned out even before they strapped him into the car. They finally managed to get him settled into the car seat and he calmed down.

However, when they arrived at their house, the crowd of friends and neighbors gathered to support them only agitated him. While they appreciated the large welcome home sign in the yard, Lindsey could hardly enjoy it while trying to calm Santana and keep his vitals in check.

Once their friends left and Lindsey and James were finally alone in their house with their two sons, she broke down. She'd prayed so long and so hard to have Santana come home, yet the son whose smile could charm his way out of any situation was gone. Throughout his stay in the hospital the doctors had warned them not to get their hopes too high for his recovery. The reality of their words hit her as she carried her son into his room. "I just want my little boy back, God," she prayed. That night she stayed close to his side, watching his vitals and applying suction as needed. Santana's first night home set the tone for every night that followed. Someone always had to stay by his side, monitoring his vitals and applying suction as needed. Lindsay and James tried to mentally prepare themselves for a lifetime of sleepless nights.

A few weeks later she learned she was pregnant with their third son.

As they settled into their new normal routine of day nurses helping with Santana's care during the day and sleepless nights spent at his side, neither Lindsey nor James were ready to give up the fight to get their son back. They traveled to Mexico for a stem cell procedure that appeared to hold out promise for children like Santana. Later they took him to a clinic in Florida for three weeks of alternative treatments. After the baby was born, the entire family spent time in California for several rounds of intense physical therapy for Santana.

After thousands of miles of travel and untold medical expenses which insurance would not cover, Lindsey and James finally came to accept that the new normal was indeed normal. This was their life. Their son was not the child he was before the accident, nor would he ever be again. Once they grieved that loss, they were free to go forward loving their son and giving him the best life they possibly could.

Santana's orthopedic surgeon was the first person to mention Ryan House to Lindsey. She'd heard talk about it in the community, and seemed to recall seeing the Care Card billboards around town, but she never thought about it as an option for Santana until Dr. Shindell told her about it "You and your family could really use Ryan House's services," he told her. "I can see the toll taking care of him is having on all of you. Ryan House is designed for families like yours. You should check it out."

Lindsey was not automatically convinced. However, since Dr. Shindell had spoken so highly of it, she decided to visit. The moment she walked in the front door, she was impressed. Staying the night in the House with Santana the first time convinced her that these people "got it." At one point during her visit she quietly went into Santana's room to check on him. He was asleep, but he was not alone. A volunteer was sitting next to him, holding his hand while he slept. "They love him like he's their own," she said to herself as she dismissed herself before she could be seen. Any qualms she might have had about leaving him alone at Ryan House disappeared.

A few months after his first stay, Lindsey and James started planning their family's annual vacation in California. Even after Santana's accident, they took him along. But after staying at Ryan House they reconsidered that decision. The long drive visibly caused him stress. While the trips were supposed to be fun for the entire family, it was clear Santana did not enjoy the hectic pace of travel. Lindsey spent so much time attending to his needs that she felt guilty for how his care took her away from their other two sons. "Let's give Santana a vacation this year," she told James. "Let's let him stay at Ryan House."

James agreed although some of their friends who also had special needs children did not. "How can you leave him out of the family activity?" they said to them. "He's part of the family, too. How can you just leave him like that?"

At first Lindsey felt a little guilty about leaving him as well, but those feelings evaporated when they pushed Santana's wheelchair through the doors. "There's our guy," Rachel, one of the nurses, said as she ran over to give Santana a hug. "I love your Mohawk."

"He seems to like it," Lindsey said.

"Looks good," Rachel replied. "We've been looking forward to your visit. I hope you're ready to have fun with us."

Several times during their vacation, Lindsey had second thoughts about leaving Santana, like every parent does when leaving their children for any time at all. However, she and James were able to give Jett and Tyree their undivided attention.

A week later when Lindsey, James and their two other sons returned, Lindsay immediately noticed Santana's Mohawk standing as tall and as straight as she always made it. Rachel walked over and handed her a book. "What's this?" Lindsay asked.

"It's a journal we kept of his week with us. We wanted you to see what Santana was up to."

Lindsay thumbed through pages filled with messages and journal entries from the care team and volunteers who worked and played with him during his stay. Photos from one of Madi's parties covered another page along with a message from Snow White who happened to visit that week. "Wow! I'm not sure who had more fun this week, you or us," she said to Santana.

"He's very popular around here," Rachel said.

"He loves attention," Lindsey said.

Rachel laughed. "We figured that out pretty quick. He got lots of it. Everyone just loves this little guy. He has a sweet spirit about him."

After his first weeklong visit, Lindsey and James made sure Santana came back often. But that was not the only contact the family had with the staff of Ryan House. At one point Santana developed a serious infection in his back. Several staff members called to check on him. They also connected Lindsey to a palliative care program as well as answered all the questions she had about it. The calls and support showed Lindsey and James that Ryan House was more than a place that cares for Santana while giving the family some much needed rest. "It's a community. It's family," Lindsey says of it.

But perhaps the best gift Ryan House ever gave the family came during the 2013 Christmas season. After one of Santana's stays at the house, Lindsey received a phone call from Julie Bank, the house Executive Director. "We would like to use one of Santana's art projects on our donor holiday cards," Julie said. "Do you think that would be okay?"

Lindsey could barely get the word "yes" out, she was so touched by the gesture. Ever since Santana's accident she and her husband had done all they could to try to "fix" him. While they had accepted who their son was now, they still missed who he had been and who he could have become. When Ryan House featured his art on their Christmas card, they did more than include Santana. They let Lindsey and James and everyone who received the card know that their son could still make a significant contribution. At Ryan House, Santana is a normal, productive child just the way he is.

Section Two: From Dream to Reality

Chapter Five

It Takes Passion

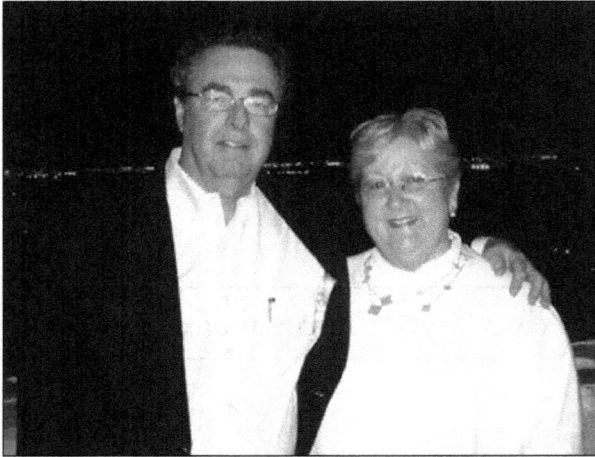

Bill and Judy Schubert

SHARON COTTOR PICKED UP THE telephone as if she'd never handled one before. For several moments she stood and stared at it. "Just make the call," she told herself. Sharon turned and walked back across the room toward her kitchen as if the phone might get up and chase her. "Just make the call," she said again. "Why are you so nervous?"

She knew the answer to her own question. She'd had this same conversation with herself several times over the past couple of days. Yet, no matter how many times Sharon picked up the phone, she could not force herself to dial the number. "How can I ask her for something like this?"

Sharon disliked asking anyone for favors, especially someone with whom she did not have a close personal relationship. And this was a huge favor. Yet she knew this was the *one* person in all of Arizona she absolutely had to call. Over the past few weeks, the same name came up every time she mentioned Jonathan and Holly's idea for building a children's hospice in Phoenix. "Have you called Judy Schubert yet?" she was asked over and over. "Oh, yes, you simply must call Judy Schubert about this. It sounds like something she would be all over."

Sharon knew they were right. That's why she, too, immediately thought of Judy Schubert when Jonathan and Holly first told her and Bob what they wanted to do. Judy had a well-earned reputation in the Valley as a woman who made things happen. She had been the driving force behind Phoenix's Ronald McDonald House twenty years earlier, and she had stayed active with them through the House's numerous expansions. Along with her husband, Bill, she'd served on the boards of many local non-profits, helping to raise hundreds of thousands of dollars over the years. A former Junior League leader and now one of the prominent members of The Board of Visitors, which was the oldest charitable organization in Arizona, Judy had strong connections to both the philanthropic and business communities. She not only knew how to get things done herself, she had close relationships with every other mover and shaker in Phoenix. If Holly and Jonathan's dream was going to get off the ground, calling Judy was the place to start. Even if she didn't want to get involved, she could point them to the people who would.

Picking up the phone one last time, Sharon let out a long sigh and punched in Judy's number. "Here we go," she said, her heart pounding.

"Hello," Judy answered.

"Judy, this is Sharon Cotton."

"Oh hi, Sharon. What can I do for you?"

"Didn't you have something to do with the Ronald McDonald House?" Sharon asked.

"Why yes I did," Judy replied. "Why do you ask?"

"My son and daughter-in-law just came back from England..." Sharon proceeded to tell Judy all about Ryan's condition, the impact it had had on the entire family and how they found a special place for rest at Helen House. "Since you were involved with the Ronald McDonald House, do you think maybe we could lean on your expertise a little? We're just getting started and not sure what to do next."

"Oh my gosh, Sharon, you may have just solved a problem for me! The

Board of Visitors and the Junior League have been talking about finding a project we can do together and this may just be it. It sounds like a wonderful idea, but let me think about it and I will get back with you."

Sharon hung up the phone and broke out in a wide grin. She didn't know it, but when Judy hung up her phone, she turned to her husband and said, "It looks like there's another house in my future."

While Sharon talked herself into calling Judy Schubert, Holly and Jonathan tried to figure out what "Going for it," was going to look like. They knew they wanted to bring a children's hospice to Phoenix but they had no illusion that they might be the people to make it happen. Ideally, they thought they might be able to find an established organization with which to partner, an organization with the size and resources to not only build a house but also to give it the credibility within the community it needed to succeed long term. George Mark Children's House in California started with a single benefactor who ultimately donated several million dollars to build and operate the House. Since the odds of that happening a second time were very slim, Holly and Diane Eckstein continued going around the Valley, meeting with people Diane thought might be interested in helping.

In the fall of 2003, Holly and Diane went to Phoenix Children's Hospital to meet Steve Schnall, the Senior Vice President and Chief Development Officer of the Phoenix Children's Hospital Foundation. Like her earlier meeting with Susan Levine, Holly found Steve liked the idea, but was noncommittal about getting personally involved. He did ask one question Holly would hear over and over through the next few years. In the middle of her presentation, Steve asked, "You know, we plan to build a Ronald McDonald House here on our campus. Aren't you talking about basically the same thing?"

"That's a good question," Holly replied, "but this is something completely different. Ronald McDonald House gives families a place to stay and function as a family while their child is in the hospital. The House we hope to build is a place families can go to any time for a respite from the rigors of caring for their special needs child while giving the child a little break from mom and dad. For the child, it's like going to Grandma's house. Our House will also offer end-of-life care for the child which is an invaluable help to the family. We plan to use a pediatric palliative care model which the Brits just call hospice although we probably won't use that word since most of us in America don't really understand what it means, not the way the Brits do. So, you see, this is very different from a Ronald McDonald House."

Steve nodded, taking it all in as Holly explained the differences. After she was finished, he gave an answer that reminded Holly of Susan Levine: "I think this is a good idea and we would be willing to help you in any way we can. But building something like this doesn't really fit into our overall mission." He then offered some good advice: "You should do a needs assessment survey before you get any further into this process. I know there are grants out there you could probably land to pay for it."

"Do you know anyone who might be able to help us with that?" Holly asked.

"Let me think about that," Steve said. "I may be able to come up with a name or two for you."

Holly left the meeting both encouraged and discouraged. "I just wish someone would catch the vision of what we want to do. I appreciate their encouragement, but I just need someone to GET it."

"I have someone else I'd like you to meet," Diane said. "Her name is Joan Lowell. She was the executive director at Hospice of the Valley before Susan and she's now at the Arizona Community Foundation. She may be able to recommend a family foundation that might be interested in funding the initial step both Steve and Susan talked about. If not, she can at least point us in the right direction."

"It's worth a shot," Holly replied.

Their meeting with Joan reminded Holly of her meetings with Susan and Steve. Joan was very polite and listened intently. But, like Steve and Susan, she didn't jump and enthusiastically exclaim, "I'm in!"

Part way through their meeting, Joan could sense Holly's disappointment with her response. Joan took Holly by the hand and said to her, "You know, sometimes it just takes a really passionate parent to make these things happen."

"I think it will take more than passion," Holly said.

"Don't sell yourself short," Joan said. "Passionate people get things done, even things that seem impossible."

Judy Schubert told Sharon she needed time to think but she didn't need much time. Something about Ryan's story resonated with her. Maybe it was the fact that she also had a son named Ryan or maybe it was the thought of all the families like the Cottors that had nowhere else to turn. Whatever it was, from the time she hung up the phone with Sharon, she knew this was her next great project.

Less than a week after their initial conversation, Judy called Sharon. "I'd like to meet Jonathan and Holly and, of course, Ryan," she said.

A day or two later, she drove over to their home. After the usual greetings and small talk, Judy got down to business. "So tell me what you want to do," she said.

Jonathan spoke up. "I think my mother has told you part of our story already, so I'll get straight to the point." He proceeded to describe Helen House and what it meant to his family. Holly brought out the flyers they'd picked up in England and handed them to Judy.

After listening for a while, Judy sat back and said, "This is really neat. To me, it sounds like we need these all over the country, not just here."

"You're absolutely right," Jonathan replied.

"Here's what I would like to do. You two are young and new in town. I'm old and I've lived here forever."

Jonathan and Holly laughed.

"Well it's true," Judy said. "I've been around here a long time and I know just about everyone in town. I've worked with most of them on one non-profit project or another. You know, I'm a western girl at heart and I love to be a pioneer. Let's figure out how to make this happen and do it."

"Ourselves?" Holly asked.

"You already are, aren't you?" Judy replied.

"Basically yes," Jonathan said. "Holly's been going around town meeting with people already. She also has a group of women she meets with here at the house who are interested in helping somehow. Of course, to me it looks like all they do is talk and agree it's a great idea and then hug."

"Jonathan!" Sharon said.

"It's true mom. If we're going to do this, let's do it. Judy, you've done big community projects. What do you think we need to do now?"

"Let me pull some people together and I'll have the two of you come and tell them what you just told me. Then we'll go from there."

The next day Judy called Judy Shannon, a member of The Board of Visitors and a long-time trustee of St. Luke's Health Initiatives. "I think I may have found our next project," she said. Judy Schubert had had a very similar conversation with another friend, Suzanne Hanson, twenty years earlier. Six years later, that conversation had turned into the first Ronald McDonald House in Phoenix. Judy Shannon did not know it yet, but this conversation was about to lead to another six year commitment.

"Okay, I'm game, what have you found?" Judy Shannon asked.

"It's another house, but this is a house for kids with life threatening conditions. You know Sharon Cottor?"

"Yes."

"Her grandson, Ryan, was born with a condition that's very serious. Just by living past his second birthday he's already beat the odds the doctors gave him when he was diagnosed. Sharon's son, Jonathan, and his wife, Holly, spent time at a House for these children and their families in England while they lived there. It was a game changer for them with Ryan. Now they want to do the same thing here."

"Wow, another house for you."

"Ironic, isn't it? After spending all those years working on the Ronald McDonald House, I never thought I'd do anything else like that again. But here I am," Judy Schubert said with a laugh. "I think this could be the perfect project for the Care Card." The Care Card is a shopping card sponsored by The Board of Visitors. Consumers purchase the card for fifty dollars, with all the proceeds going to a local charity selected by The BOV. Shoppers may then use the card at hundreds of participating retailers and restaurants in the

Phoenix Metropolitan area to receive a twenty percent discount on all full price purchases made during the last ten days of October. Judy Schubert borrowed the idea from Texas. The Card caught on quickly. Soon, The BOV was donating six figure amounts from the card to charity each year.

"I'm going to have a meeting with a few BOV women about it in the next week or two," Judy Schubert continued. "I'm also thinking of inviting some of the Junior League leaders[4]. I've always wanted to find something the two of us could do together, especially since all of us in BOV were once Junior League."

"Until we got too old," Judy Shannon laughed.

"Well there's that," Judy Schubert replied.

A couple of weeks later, Jonathan and Holly walked into Judy Schubert's living room. Bob and Sharon came along for moral support. Unlike her earlier meeting with Susan Levine, Holly was not at all nervous. More than anything, she and Jonathan were both excited. "I think we're finally getting some traction," Jonathan said on their drive over. "We need to get the community to buy into what we want to do, and I think it starts tonight."

"I hope so," Holly said.

When they walked into the room, Judy immediately took them around the room, introducing them individually to several of the women in attendance. She then introduced the two of them to the group. "I am excited for all of you to get to hear what Jonathan and Holly have to say," she said. "When I first heard their story, my heart went out to them. We both have sons named Ryan, after all. But I think they have a very good idea for something we need here in the Valley. We need these all over the country, not just here. But everything has to start somewhere, so it might as well be here. Jonathan, why don't you tell us what you have in mind?"

Jonathan stood and told their story of Ryan's diagnosis, the toll his illness took upon the entire family, all leading up to their experience at Helen House. "This will give you an idea of what we hope to build," he said as he popped a Helen House VHS cassette into the tape deck. He'd ordered it from England

---

4 The Junior League is a volunteer organization of women dedicated to making an impact in their community.

not long after reading the book, "A House Called Helen."

After his presentation, Judy spoke up. "For years, The Board of Visitors has raised funds for charities connected to the medical needs of our community. But with so many of the hospitals now operated by for-profit companies, a lot of the places with whom we used to work are no longer options for us. But this house is exactly the kind of work we need to be involved in. I also think this is the kind of project both The BOV and Junior League can get behind. If we work together, we can make this happen. A lot of people have tried to build a 'Helen House' here in the United States but no one has pulled it off, at least not like this. I plan on us being the first. Besides, I like the idea of building something, don't you?"

Judy sparked a spirited conversation that lit up the room. No one questioned the idea. Everyone picked up on Judy's lead and started discussing how they could pull this off.

The response in the room overwhelmed Holly. For months she'd talked to one person after another, trying to find someone to champion this cause in the community. She hoped to find someone who might share her passion and want this house to happen just as badly as she did. Watching Judy speak, she knew she'd finally found a champion. She knew they were now truly on their way.

After the meeting broke up Judy walked Sharon to the door. "Thank you so much for doing this," Sharon said. "I cannot tell you how much this means to me and to my family."

"Thank you for calling me and telling me about this. I tell you, we are going to build this house and when we do, we'll call it Ryan House!"

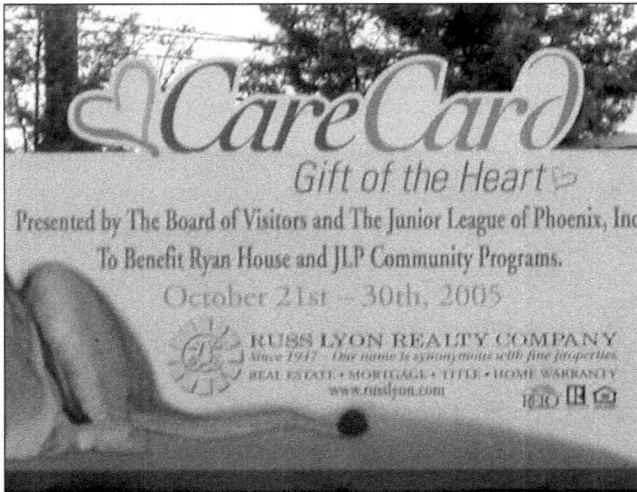

Billboard in Central Phoenix promoting the
"Care Card" to benefit Ryan House

Chapter Six

The Game Plan

NOT LONG AFTER HOLLY AND Diane's meeting with Steve Schnall of Phoenix Children's Hospital, he called and made good on his promise to recommend someone who could help the Cottors secure a grant for the needs assessment survey. Rachel Oesterle had recently started her own business as a consultant to non-profit organizations. She helped groups evaluate their overall structure and operations, improving their ability both to fulfill their mission and insure their long term sustainability. Prior to starting her own firm, Rachel spent fourteen years as executive director of Aid to Adoption of Special Kids. Her work with that organization earned her an "Angel of Arizona" award for her leadership in the foster care and adoption arena. Working with at risk children also made her very sensitive to the needs of families like Holly and Jonathan's.

The Cottors presented a unique situation to Rachel. With little more than a commitment to "go for it," their "organization" had yet to organize. They didn't even have a formal name for what they wanted to do.

Rachel and Holly hit it off from the start. Not long after being introduced by Steve, Rachel became part of Holly's "kitchen cabinet" of women interested in building a children's hospice in Phoenix. Others in the group included Nancy White and Cheryl Thomas, both of whom worked for Hospice of the Valley's fund development, and Leslie Jaap-Propstra, a retired IBM Executive. Rachel listened closely to the group's ideas. The more she listened, the more convinced she became that she could help the Cottors reach their goal.

One afternoon after most of the kitchen cabinet members had left, Rachel approached Holly. "I think it is time we start formalizing the ideas being thrown out into a step-by-step action plan."

"I was hoping you would say that," Holly replied. "I know we have a lot of good ideas but they're all so scattered. I don't know what to do first."

"You have the most important part of the equation," Rachel said. "You have a very clear vision of what you want to accomplish. A lot of the organizations with whom I work have either never had a clear vision or they lost it somewhere along the way. That makes it hard for them to get anywhere. But when you know where you want to go, figuring out how to get there is the easy part."

"So where do we start?" Holly asked.

Over the next few months, Holly and Rachel met together at the Cottors' dining room table and hammered out the answer to that question. They tried to meet at least once a week, but sometimes life as the mother of two young sons got in Holly's way. Jonathan pitched in with the boys as much as he could, but there were times Ryan and Ethan just needed their mom. When that happened, her strategy sessions with Rachel went on the back burner. More than once during this time Jonathan asked, "What do you need me to do? I want to get involved with this as well."

"I've got it," Holly always answered. "I know you have the entrepreneurial mind and business background, not to mention the spirit and passion we need to succeed, but I'd like to try and take this as far as I can before you jump in. I hope you can understand."

"Of course," Jonathan replied, "but know I am always here for you whenever you need me."

Even with the delays, Holly and Rachel's plan began to take shape. They structured everything around five goals.[5] First on the list was the goal to complete a formal business plan. As Rachel explained it to Holly, the House they hoped to build had to become a business long before they even broke ground. Their first phase objectives included formulating a budget, securing 501(c)(3) status as a bona fide non-profit organization, creating a board of directors and conducting a full feasibility study to discover whether a children's hospice could survive long term in Phoenix.

Once they created a business plan, they could create a formal services plan. In short, this plan would define what the house would do and be. Their

5 See Appendix A

third goal focused on fundraising, both for the capital campaign to build Ryan House as well as a comprehensive fundraising program to support the House long term.

Their fourth goal concentrated on establishing their proposed children's hospice within the Arizona community. Basically, they wanted to find a way to get the community to buy into a children's hospice to such a degree that the community as a whole would never let it close its doors. Before the community could buy into the children's hospice, it needed to understand it. Both Rachel and Holly knew it would be a challenge to create awareness of something that only now existed as an idea but they could not wait until the house was built to start promoting it. They made one of their objectives creating a brand that people could see even before the first shovel full of dirt was moved.

Finally, their plan set a goal of creating a plan for the operations of Ryan House, including how it would serve the children and families for whom it was to be built. "It seems a little odd that the one thing we really want to do is last on our list," Holly said as she typed the goal out.

"But if we don't reach our first four goals, we'll never make it to the last one," Rachel replied. "This is our destination, this is where we want to arrive. The destination always comes last, not first."

While Holly and Rachel worked on their strategic goals, Judy Schubert also got busy. Jonathan gave her a copy of "A House Called Helen," which she devoured. Judy, in turn, gave Holly a copy of the bylaws to the Ronald McDonald House which she helped put together. "We started from scratch with that one, too," Judy told them. "A few Ronald McDonald Houses existed in other parts of the country, but that only gave us name recognition and some credibility when we started talking about doing it here. We still had to get the community to buy into it which is what we have to do now."

The first step toward community buy-in was to pull together in one place as many people as possible from the pediatric medical community, hospice community and the families with children with life threatening conditions. Hospice of the Valley provided a conference room for them to use and also promoted the event with their employees. Holly had built relationships with several people at HOV and invited several personally to attend. Judy knew the key people in the nonprofit community and invited those she thought might be receptive to this project. Her husband, Bill, was involved with the board of St. Joseph's Hospital which extended invites to people within the medical community. Holly and Jonathan also had several contacts within the medical community because of Ryan's care, including physical therapists, nurses and pediatricians. They invited everyone they thought might be willing to listen to their idea.

Dr. David Hirsch accepted their invitation. His practice was the leading pediatric office in Phoenix specializing in caring for children with chronic, congenital, and life limiting conditions and diseases. In the late 1990's, Hospice of the Valley approached him about starting a pediatric team for their child hospice patients. Since he treated so many children with life threatening conditions already, he knew the challenges these families faced. He accepted HOV's offer as a logical extension of his care for his patients. At the time, children in need of hospice stayed at one of HOV's adult facilities. However, Dr. Hirsch had always dreamed of having a pediatric facility that could also provide palliative as well as end-of-life care. When he heard about the Cottors' idea, he thought this might just be the ticket.

Even though at this point in the process this project was Holly's thing, both she and Jonathan spoke at this first community meeting. Holly began by telling the story of Ryan's diagnosis and the impact his condition had made on their entire family. Jonathan picked up the story and talked about Helen House. "It was the first children's hospice in the world but now they've spread all over the UK" With tears now streaming down his face, he added, "We only had a chance to stay a few times and I don't know how we'll survive without it. That's why we want to pioneer the British children's hospice model right here in Phoenix." He then showed the video he had shown Judy Schubert a few months earlier.

"So what do you think?" Jonathan asked the group. Watching Jonathan, Holly thought, *it's time now for him to really get involved.*

David Hirsch spoke up. "Most of you know of my involvement with

Hospice of the Valley in starting pediatric hospice care here in Phoenix. Jonathan, Holly, I have to tell you that what you've described here is exactly what I've always hoped to see children's hospice become. I've wanted to see a children's hospice facility for a very long time."

Others spoke up, agreeing on the need. However, one question kept coming up over and over. "Do we have to call it a children's *hospice*?"

"But that's what it is," Jonathan replied.

"I know, but I'm afraid if we went into the community talking about a hospice for children, people would get the wrong idea. I know I probably shouldn't say this, considering where we are, but for most people, hospice means the end. And what you are describing here is definitely not the end for these children."

"I think I can help," Dr. Hirsch spoke up. "My practice specializes in caring for exactly the kind of children this facility would help. Most of these families will probably resist using the term 'hospice' in connection with their children. However, we're actually talking about palliative care which is a word all of these families know and embrace. I also think they would respond to the idea of a place that offers respite care. From my experience, all of these families operate on the edge of exhaustion. I believe they will respond very positively to an emphasis on a place where they can actually rest and refresh."

The conversation continued. Most agreed with Dr. Hirsch. As the meeting began to wind down, Jonathan suddenly realized that the talk had long since stopped focusing on whether or not this house was needed. Instead, all the participants discussed the particulars as if building it was already a foregone conclusion. He glanced over at Holly. The look on her face told him she had the same realization. *This is really going to happen!* he thought to himself. *Oh my God. It is now just a question of when, not if.*

"So, what are you going to call this house you want to build?" someone asked.

"We haven't really gotten that far," Holly replied.

Judy Schubert chimed in. "I think it is only natural that it be called Ryan House. Helen House was named after the little girl whose illness prompted the creation of that house. If it weren't for Ryan, we wouldn't be having this conversation right now."

Several other people spoke up, saying the same thing. Before the meeting was over, several even spoke of it as Ryan House.

"But this is for all the families in the community who have children with life limiting conditions," Jonathan objected, "not just ours."

"Of course," came the reply, "but we have to call it something. I think Ryan House captures what we want to do here."

Dr. Hirsch added one more thought before the meeting ended. "The facility we're discussing here tonight does not easily fit into any existing models in our community. I think as we go forward from here we need to keep this independent from any of the area hospitals or even Hospice of the Valley. I am afraid the moment one of the other organizations takes this project on, they will reshape it to fit the existing model of what they already do. Now don't get me wrong. I have worked in and with all of the hospitals and organizations I'm talking about. I respect them and their work. But this project is so different I really think the only way to achieve the goals Jonathan and Holly have so eloquently described is to make it a completely independent organization."

After the meeting broke up, Holly approached Dr. Hirsch. "I so appreciate your input tonight. I cannot tell you how much it meant to us."

"Like I said, I've always wanted to see something like this here in Phoenix. I think there's a real need here," he replied. "I'd heard a little about the two of you before tonight. You know, I am a colleague of Jonathan's parents and have known them and their work for nearly thirty years."

"I didn't realize that," Holly said. "Phoenix really is just a small town masquerading as a big city, isn't it?"

Dr. Hirsch laughed. "It certainly seems that way sometimes."

Holly then asked a question without hesitation. "Would you be willing to join a group with whom I meet on a regular basis to help shape this idea?"

"Like a steering committee?" he replied.

"Yes. A steering committee," Holly said.

"Certainly. Thank you for asking."

Jonathan and Holly returned home after the meeting emotionally drained but ecstatic. "So what do you think?" Holly asked Jonathan.

"I think this is happening. The momentum and enthusiasm in the room tonight was amazing."

"I am blown away by it," Holly replied.

"So, what now?" Jonathan asked.

"We develop the business plan," Holly said, "secure 501(c)(3) status, create a board of directors and go from there.

"Business is what I do," Jonathan said. "Why don't you let me take part of that and run with it?"

"That's a good idea."

"Great. So tomorrow I will contact the attorney Debbie Shumway recommended from Hospice of the Valley and find out what we have to do to get non-profit status. I also think we should go ahead and incorporate 'Ryan House.'"

"Wow! I never imagined naming this after Ryan," Holly said. She paused and fought back tears. Finally she said, "I just hope he lives long enough to see it."

The next day Jonathan wrote a check for $700 to incorporate Ryan House. The idea they'd talked about for over a year now had a name and a legal entity. It also had zero dollars in the bank. Even so, they were on their way.

Around that same time, Jonathan and Holly wrote another check, this one to Helen House. They attached a letter, telling Sister Frances, the Founder and a Trustee, how much the house meant to them during their time in England. "We're trying to build a house modeled after yours here in Arizona," they wrote. "We know others have tried before, but we are determined to see this through to completion. Thank you again for all you have done for our family."

A few weeks later a letter arrived in the mail with a London postmark. Inside, the letter on Helen House stationary said:

Dear Jonathan, Holly, Ethan and Ryan,
Thank you so much for your wonderful letter telling us of your exciting plans for Ryan House. It does not need me to tell you what a lot of

hard work lies ahead, but if anyone can succeed I know you will!

Please be assured of our ongoing support and prayers and remember that if there is anything at all we can ever do to help, you have only to let us know. Thank you so much for the most generous gift – so good of you when you need every penny for your own project.

Everyone here joins me in sending you our love and all possible good wishes.

God bless you.
Yours most sincerely,

Frances
Sister Frances Dominica
Founder and Trustee

Jonathan looked up at Holly after reading the letter. "Well that seals it, doesn't it?"

"What do you mean?" Holly said.

"We *have* to see this through to the end now. I'm not letting Sister Frances down. Are you?"

Holly laughed. "No, I guess not."

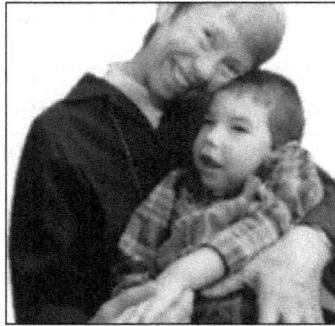

Sister Frances

Donavan

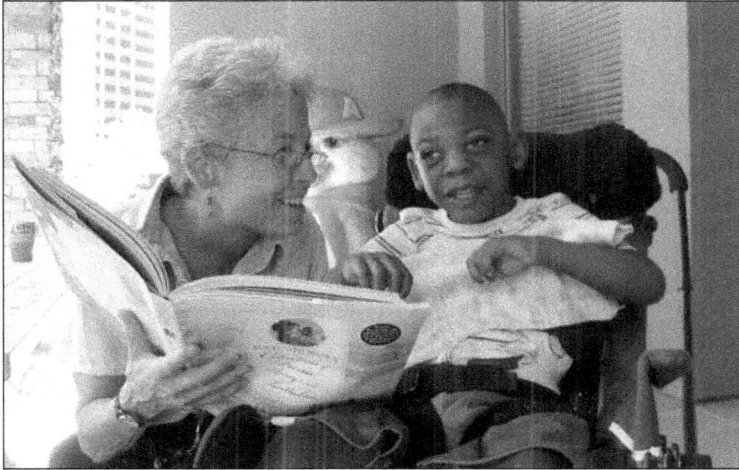

Donavan and Jo enjoy reading on the patio at Ryan House

Toya walked slowly to the door of Donavan's room. She didn't want to take a chance of her son hearing her. If he heard her voice, he would want her and not Kasia. Toya had watched the two of them from afar throughout the evening. It was their first night ever at Ryan House. Every family must stay in one of the family suites on their first stay at the House before they can leave a child at the house alone. Tonight, Toya wouldn't have it any other way. Aside from his stays at Phoenix Children's Hospital, she'd never been apart from Donavan overnight. While she knew he was in good hands, she had to make sure.

All moms are protective of their children, but Toya is even more so. Donavan is a miracle child. Born after only twenty four weeks, he came into the world weighing one pound, eleven ounces. His twin brother contracted an infection and died when he was only five days old, but Donavan kept on fighting. He spent the first five months of his life in the NICU. During that time the doctors caring for him broke the news to Toya that her son had cerebral palsy with quadriplegic impairment. He would never walk or talk or do any of the things of which Toya imagined she would do with her child when she found out she was pregnant. Nor could Donavan eat on his own, which necessitated the hospital inserting a G-tube.

In spite of his difficulties, Donavan's personality shone from the time he was an infant. He captured the heart of everyone who met him with his infectious smile. Though legally blind, he never missed anything that happened around him. And though he couldn't speak, he found ways to let you know what he wanted.

Donavan was truly a miracle child, but caring for him was not easy for Toya. A single mom, her seventy plus year old mother was her only back up for his care, which is extensive. He depended on her for everything. Not that she minded. Even so, getting up with Donavan two or three times a night, every night, along with caring for him in the same way one must care for a newborn eventually took its toll.

That is why Toya immediately made an appointment to visit Ryan House after a friend told her about it. Two weeks later when she and Donavan (five years old), first arrived at Ryan House for their overnight stay, she went over her "Donavan must-do" list two or three times with the staff. Even though she was just down the hall in one of the Ryan House family suites, Toya was apprehensive about letting someone take over for her for even one night – that's why she kept sneaking out of her room and peaking in on him. Earlier in the evening she'd watched him sit in wonder in the sensory room as music played and other children laughed and played. Donavan loved being around other children almost as much as he loved music. He didn't get many chances to interact with other children at home. This place was different.

Toya also watched him in the music room as Jamie, a volunteer, placed a maraca in his hand. "You can play along," Jamie said as she helped Donavan shake the maraca. He broke out in a big grin. Toya loved to see her son smile.

His fun day wore him out. Kasia, one of the certified nurse assistants on staff at Ryan House, bathed him and dressed him for bed while Toya went back to her room and dove into a book. Although she loved to read, she hadn't had much time for it since Donavan was born. The family suite was set back from the main hall just far enough to make it extra quiet. The room itself had the look and feel of a nice hotel room. For a moment, Toya lost herself in her book and forgot where she was. Her eyes started growing heavy, but a thought hit her that woke her right up: Donavan! I have to check on Donavan.

That thought is what brought her back into the hall just outside of her son's room. From inside she heard the sound of soft humming. Careful not to make a sound, she crept closer. Her first thought as she peaked inside was, Why is his bed empty? Then she looked over toward the corner of the room. Kasia sat in a chair with Donavan cuddled up on her lap. As she rocked back and forth, Kasia softly sang a lullaby to Donavan. He appeared to be completely at peace.

Toya struggled to hold herself together. The sight of a complete stranger (at least a stranger up until a few hours earlier) loving her son, overwhelmed her. Any qualms she had about Ryan House disappeared. She went back to her room and her book. The next thing she knew, light was streaming in her window. This was her first full, uninterrupted night of sleep in so long that she'd forgotten what real rest felt like.

Immediately, Toya's thoughts turned to her son. She went back to his room to check on him. This time she was not afraid to let him hear her voice. Rachel, one of the staff nurses, was just leaving his room as Toya walked up. "How is my little man this morning?" Toya asked.

"Still sleeping," Rachel said.

Toya could not believe her ears. Donavan always woke up very, very early. She looked up at the clock. It was just past seven. "Are you sure?" Toya asked.

"I just left him. Everything looks good. He's sleeping like a baby."

"Wow. He never sleeps this late at home." Toya went back to her room and took a long, hot shower. When she returned to Donavan's room an hour or so later, he was up and dressed. "What do you have planned for the day?" Rachel asked.

"Nothing really. I thought I might just hang out here for a while and read or watch a movie before the two of us go home this afternoon," Toya replied.

"Have you ever taken Donavan swimming?" Rachel said.

"One time, but he didn't like the cold water."

"The two of you should try our hydrotherapy room. I think Donavan would respond very well to it. The pool is designed for the children but parents can get in with them."

"I'm not so sure," Toya said with that protective mother tone.

"The water is very warm and you won't be alone with him unless you just want to be. I or one of the other staff members can help you and even get in the water with the two of you if you would like," Rachel reassured her.

"I don't know," Toya replied. "I guess we could take a look at it and see."

A short time later Toya found herself sitting on the pool steps, holding her son. He could not stop smiling. Rachel and a CNA were also in the water helping Toya support Donavan. Toya took his hand and splashed it in the water. "How does that feel, baby? Do you like that?" He clearly did. She lowered him a little more into the water so that his legs could swing free of her. He started kicking hard, splashing water around her. At first she was afraid he might feel panicked but when he resisted her attempts to pull him back onto her lap she could tell he was just having fun. Toya looked over at Rachel with tears in her eyes. "I don't get many moments like this with my son," she said. "Thank you for suggesting this."

After their first visit, Toya felt very comfortable leaving Donavan by himself at Ryan House. Although she did not spend the night there again, she still returned on a regular basis. For her, Ryan House was more than a place for a respite stay for her son. She connected with the staff which only made sense. Moms love those who love their children and Toya found all the staff and volunteers at Ryan House continually pouring love on Donavan. He enjoyed staying at the House as well. Donavan loved being around other children. At Ryan House, there were always other children playing and making noise. He enjoyed taking it all in. But the House wasn't just for him.

Toya discovered how much Ryan House cared for her one Mother's Day. As a single mom of a special needs, non-communicative child, Mother's Day was usually a little lonely. However, one Mother's Day she received an invitation to come to an event at Ryan House. She and Donavan had attended several special events at the House over the years, including Easter egg hunts and movie nights. But this event was designed for Toya, not her son.

When Toya arrived she discovered she was one of five single moms invited to a Mother's Day brunch. The living room had been transformed just for them. The brunch buffet included fruits and pastries. Gift bags lined one table, one for each of them. Inside the bag, Toya found a variety of makeup and lip gloss. A makeup clinician was on hand to give each mom a mini makeover, doing their makeup and their hair. A young couple was also there. Toya learned their child had recently died at Ryan House. The care and support they received meant so much to them that they wanted to give something back. This was their chance. The two were photographers. They took photographs of the moms with their kids, and gave each mother a disk with the photos. Ryan House also gave each mom a framed picture.

Today, Toya takes advantage of Ryan House at least once a quarter. She never leaves Donavan for more than a few days. He's a momma's boy who doesn't like being away from his mother for long. But they both need small breaks from one another, just like any other parent and child. Toya didn't know how she kept going before Ryan House came into her life. Parents in her situation do not realize how stressed and tired they've become until they have a moment to step away and recharge. Without that break, many snap or just give out. Toya understands how that could happen. During her first visit she realized just how exhausted she had become. Now the small breaks from the demands of caring for her son around the clock give her the strength she needs to carry on. After a stay at Ryan House she comes home recharged, ready to confront whatever lies ahead of the two of them.

Chapter Seven

At the Intersection of First and Merrell

AFTER HER EXPERIENCE BUILDING THE first Ronald McDonald House in Phoenix, Judy Schubert knew it was never too early to start scouting locations for her newest project. Her search took her not to a place, but a name: Linda Hunt, the CEO of St. Joseph's Hospital and Medical Center in the heart of Phoenix. Judy's husband, Bill, served on the hospital's foundation board of directors and Judy had been very involved with the hospital in a variety of capacities through the years. But that wasn't why Judy thought of Linda and St. Joseph's. Judy had watched as St. Joseph's provided millions of dollars in free care to those who could not afford to go to the doctor or stay in a hospital. That kind of community mindedness was key if a place like Ryan House was going to succeed. Linda also demonstrated strong leadership and the willingness to make decisions on her own without having to consult scores of advisers when she believed in a course of action.

On top of all of that, Judy kept driving past an empty lot on St. Joseph's complex that looked like the perfect location. Situated in the middle of the city one block from Phoenix's new light rail system, the location looked perfect. Families could have access to all the food and entertainment options downtown Phoenix offered. Moms and dads staying in the family suites could rest assured that their child was receiving excellent care while they jumped on the train and headed off to a Diamondbacks baseball game or a Suns basketball game without having to worry about parking. Judy also thought it wise to have Ryan House near a hospital emergency room, just in case.

Her only hesitation came from Dr. Hirsch's words in the first community meeting. *Ryan House needed to stay independent*, he'd said more than once. Placing the House on St. Joseph's campus might give the impression that this was little more than an extension of the hospital. Another hospital in town had already offered to place Ryan House inside an existing wing of the hospital. No one on the steering committee thought that was a good idea. Neither did

Judy. However, her experience with the Ronald McDonald House taught her a lot about the politics within the local medical community. If they rejected one offer and then turned around and put Ryan House on the campus of another hospital, feelings would be hurt and the ensuing controversy could keep the community as a whole from buying into the House. *But these kids are more important than silly politics,* Judy kept telling herself. *If this is where the House needs to be, it is where it needs to be, whether it is next to St. Joseph's hospital or the city zoo.* Judy and Jonathan had already looked at other locations, and nothing compared to the empty lot on St. Joseph's campus.

"I think it is the perfect spot," Judy told her husband, Bill. "You're on the foundation board, what do you think?"

"I think we're going to build a parking complex on that piece of ground," he said.

"A parking garage? People can park anywhere. Building a special place for these kids is a much better use of that land. Don't you agree?"

Bill didn't argue the point. He knew better.

A few weeks later, Judy invited Linda to meet her for breakfast. She also invited Holly and Jonathan and their two boys to come along. When Ryan came rolling up in his chair, Linda was struck by the sight of such a small boy navigating so well. "You're a pretty good driver," she said to Ryan.

He grinned.

"You should see the holes he's put in the walls at home," Ethan said with that big brother tone that lets his little brother know he thinks he's a dork.

Jonathan ignored the remark and turned to Linda. "Anyway, thank you for meeting with us this morning," he said. He then shared some of his family's story. "Holly and I are fortunate to have such a supportive family, but they are not always comfortable helping with the type of care that Ryan needs; especially when he's sick. It can be incredibly technical and very difficult for people with no caregiving background to pull off. That means we can't just drop the boys off at my 'parents' house and take off for the weekend."

"As you well know from the people who come in and out of your hospital, there are lots of families like ours out there," Holly chimed in. "Many have far greater needs. Some families we know are almost like 'invisible families.' Their child's care is so consuming that they never leave home. They rarely go on vacations, if at all. Their other children suffer because they don't get the attention they need. That's why Ryan House is so desperately needed. It will be a place where these families can come for respite, then go back home and have the strength to keep doing what they have to do."

"So what do you think, Linda?" Judy asked.

"I think it sounds wonderful but the site you asked me about when you first called is not available. We're planning to put another hospital building there," Linda said.

Judy was surprised, but undaunted. "But that spot is perfect."

"That's why we're going to put a new building on it. I tell you what. Let me think this through and I will get back with you."

Judy gave Linda a copy of "A House Called Helen" before she left. Linda promised to read it, a promise she immediately kept. The idea of a children's hospice struck her as a genuine need. After reading the book, she was even more convinced.

Not long after their breakfast meeting, Linda and her husband flew to London for a board meeting she chairs. While she was there, she called Helen House. Soon she had Sister Frances on the line. Linda explained who she was and mentioned the Ryan House project. "I'd like to come out and take a look around, if that is all right with you," she said.

"Certainly. We would love to have you," Sister Frances replied.

The next day, Linda, her husband and a photographer on her team boarded a train and headed off to Oxford. They spent the day at Helen House talking with the staff, meeting families and taking photographs. By the time they left, Linda was hooked. "We have to make this happen," she told her husband on the trip back to their hotel.

When Linda returned to Phoenix, she called Judy Schubert. "Judy, I made a little side trip while I was in London," she said.

"And...?" Judy asked.

"And we *will* find a way to make Ryan House happen. I spent a day talking with the families and staff at Helen House. We have to create our own version of that here."

Judy could hardly contain her excitement. She felt like jumping up and down.

"Here's what I would like to do," Linda continued, "I have a piece of land on the corner of First and Merrell that I think will work for you. I can't give it away but I can probably convince my board to lease it to you long term so that you can build on it. Why don't you take a look at it and let me know if it will work for you size-wise with what you want to build."

Judy started calculating costs in her head. She knew what prime property in the heart of Phoenix went for. "What kind of lease do you have in mind?"

"I don't know. How does a fifty year lease for say, a dollar a year sound?"

"I think we could probably find the money to make that happen," Judy said with a laugh.

"Don't worry about the rent. I will take care of that," Linda said. And she did. The actual lease turned out to be for sixty years at a dollar a year. Linda wrote the check for $60 to cover it.

The next day, Judy and Jonathan drove over to the property to take a look at it. They found an oddly shaped dirt lot with a parking garage on one side and a bank building on the other. "I don't know, Judy," Jonathan said, "it really isn't what I envisioned. Helen House had such large, spacious gardens. There's no room for that here. The steering committee had also talked about having a pool for the families to use while they are staying here. A decent sized pool would take the entire lot."

"I know it might not be exactly what you had envisioned," Judy replied, "but try to see it for what it is. A light rail station is going to be a block east of here which will be good for families who stay at the house. We're close to shopping and lots of restaurants. And St. Joe's is right down the street, which should set 'families' minds at ease when it comes to leaving their children here."

"Yeah, well, I don't know," Jonathan said.

"Let's bring in an architect and see what he can come up with and go from there," Judy said. "If we can make it work, this is three-quarters of a million dollars we don't have to raise for land."

"I do like the location. Okay, let's see what the architects can come up with," Jonathan concluded.

While Judy recruited Clint Miller, of Miller Associates, to develop the initial architectural site plan, Linda went to bat for Ryan House with her board of directors. The hospital's long range facilities plan called for expanding a parking garage onto the property on which Linda wanted to place Ryan House. Changing those plans meant calling in her team of strategic planners and architects to see how they could meet their projected parking needs without this one piece of land.

"Because of its odd shape, the property at First and Merrell is going to be a tough fit whatever we do with it," Linda said. "We probably need to move these planned parking spaces elsewhere even without Ryan House. In all likelihood we're never going to be able to use this land effectively anyway," she explained in their meetings. The team agreed. She'd cleared her first hurdle.

Next she had to go to the hospital sponsors. St. Joseph's Medical Center was then part of Catholic Health Care West, a ministry of the Sisters of Mercy, one of the oldest Catholic women's organizations in the world with roots going back to Catherine McAuley, an Irish laywoman who founded the movement in Dublin in 1827. Linda referred to the Sisters' ministry statement, which was also the hospital's ministry statement. The statement pledged to care for the needs of the poor, sick and under served. "These children and their families are truly under served," Linda explained. She went on to show how the mission of Ryan House fit into the overall mission of the Sisters. Referring to data she'd pulled from St. Joseph's pediatric units, she explained how hundreds of the hospital's current and former patients would benefit from Ryan House.

When the Sisters of Mercy signed off on Linda's plan, she still had one more hurdle. Even though St. Joseph's Medical Center had its own board of directors, and even though it was part of Catholic Health Care West, ultimately the hospital and all its property were owned by the Catholic Church.

Therefore, before Linda could lease any of their land to Ryan House, she had to receive approval from the Vatican. She wrote a letter, explaining what she wanted to do and why. In it she included much of the same data she'd presented to the Sisters. Months went by without a response. Finally, the Vatican approved her plan.

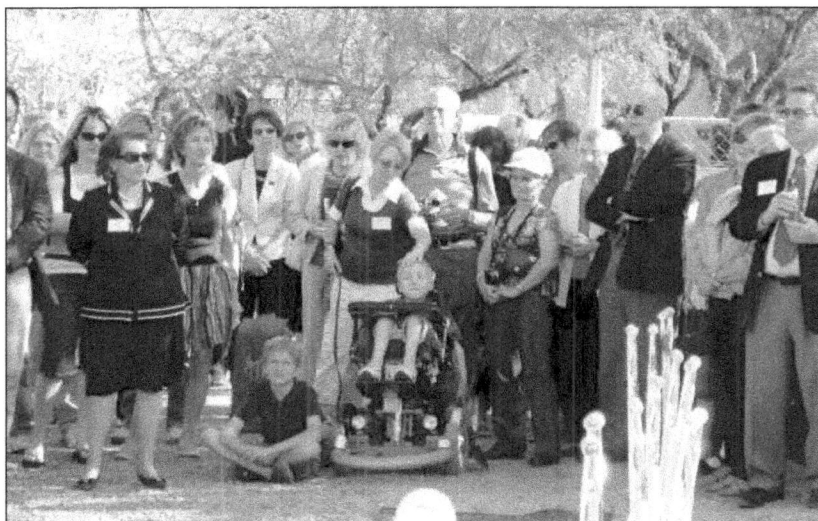

Linda Hunt (front left), Ryan and Holly (center), and Bill Schubert (front right) at ceremonial ground breaking dedication

The loosely formed Ryan House steering committee that met in the Cottor's dining room or Diane Eckstein's living room was formalized into a bonafide board of directors. Their first meeting, also held in Diane's living room, took up the question of whether or not the proposed piece of land would work for the house they envisioned. Jonathan, who was elected to serve as the board's first chair, still had serious reservations about the property. However, he started to warm up to it when he saw the architect's initial drawings. While the house still seemed a little small after also trying to squeeze both a small pool and parking spaces onto the land, Linda alleviated that concern. "We will provide parking in our lot next door," she explained. "You don't need to waste any space for that. And as for the pool, our master plan calls for an aquatic center for therapy across the street from Ryan House. Your families will have carte blanche access to it any time they want."

Clint Miller went back to the drawing board and revised his plans taking advantage of the added space. When he came back with his new drawings, the board knew they'd found a home for Ryan House. The proposed 14,000 square foot design included all the bedrooms, family suites and therapy rooms the house needed. Mr. Miller had even squeezed in garden spaces outside. "That's it!" Jonathan said, "It is exactly what we dreamt of building."

The board of directors agreed. One of their first moves was signing off on the site at First and Merrell.

Ryan House now had a place to call home.

More than that, the property and all Linda had to go through to win approval for Ryan House to use it gave the project a level of credibility it did not have before. Not only did they have a physical site, but one of the largest and most respected medical centers in Arizona had endorsed the plan in a decisive way. Ryan House was no longer just an idea. Now it seemed it was only a matter of time before they broke ground. First, however, there was the question of raising a few million dollars to build and sustain the house, seven million, to be exact. But more than raising money, the Board now faced the task of showing the community as a whole how badly Ryan House was needed. Once the community bought in, the rest would surely fall into place.

Chapter Eight

Magic

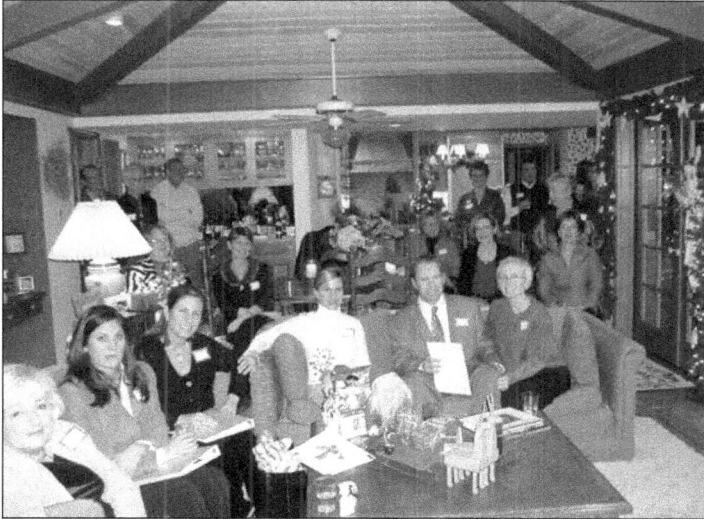

The original Board of Directors' year-end holiday
meeting at the Schubert's home

RYAN HOUSE STARTED OUT AS little more than a "Wouldn't it be nice?" that kept coming up in Holly's conversations with one person after another. Then Diane Eckstein replied, "Well, why not?" For a time it appeared the idea might stall there. Holly and Diane met with one community leader after another hoping to find someone who would "GET!" the vision and catch their passion, to no avail. At first they heard lots of "That's a nice idea, I wish you well, but it's not really something we do."

Then Judy Schubert came along. She GOT it in a big, big way. Judy Shannon and Susan Palmer-Hunter also got it. So did Dr. David Hirsch, and Rachel Osterle. When Judy, Judy and Susan shared the idea with The Board of Visitors and the Junior League of Phoenix – both organizations got it. Before long, passion for Ryan House spread as more and more people got behind the project. It was, as one person after another described it, *magic*, although, in the world of building a non-profit from the ground up, magic is just another word for a lot of hard work done passionately.

The initial board of directors came together in this way. Jan Johnson, a consultant hired by the board two years in, called this her miracle board because it defied the usual, time proven formula for building a non-profit founding board of directors. Normally, a board is formed only after a feasibility study is completed. The study evaluates whether or not the proposed project is needed and whether the community will support it long term. The study normally discovers potential donors and board members with connections to even more donors. A board then forms and the organization proceeds from there.

Ryan House flipped the process upside down. The group that became the board had already committed to going forward before the first potential donor was ever identified. Only then did the board commission a feasibility study. The first donation didn't follow the normal pattern either. The Cottors scheduled a family ski trip with Holly's parents. They were invited to stay with Budd and Judi at the home of some close friends. Fueled by hours of sharing stories of the Cottor family's challenges, tears, accomplishments and dreams, the Busche's friends were anxious to meet Ethan and Ryan and hear more from Holly and Jonathan personally. Neither Holly nor Jonathan even mentioned needing money for the project. A financial appeal was the furthest thing from their minds. They were there to ski and relax with family and friends. After listening to the two of them share passionately about starting a place for respite for families like theirs, the friends wanted to support them and be a part of making the house become a reality. No one needed to ask; they got it. Holly and Jonathan were both overwhelmed when Holly received a donation check for $10,000 in the mail the following week!

Many of the early board members committed to serve in the same way. They received a formal invitation, but only after it was clear to all that they were already part of the board of directors which had not yet formally been organized. Diane Eckstein and Judy Schubert became part of the board in that way. When discussions finally got around to creating an actual board, they were natural additions. All those involved also assumed that either Holly or Jonathan would chair the board. The two of them decided Jonathan was a better fit because of his business background although Holly remained just as involved as ever. Judy Shannon was also a natural fit on the board. She'd worked with Judy Schubert on projects like this in the past. She also served on The Board of Visitors, which already was becoming more and more invested in Ryan House. Another BOV member, Susan Palmer-Hunter, was invited to serve on the board. She and Judy Schubert, along with Susie Chester, had worked together on bringing the Care Card to Phoenix. Susan, like Judy, was eager to tackle another house.

The Junior League of Phoenix had also committed to Ryan House through the Care Card. Therefore, it only seemed natural for its president, Tara Kilby, to come onto the Ryan House board. Two other Junior League members, Patty Taylor and Kris Scardello, joined soon after, as did former Junior League president Faye Tait. All were experienced fundraisers with a heart for area non-profits. Jonathan rounded out the board by inviting a family friend and financial planner, Chuck Scott, to join as treasurer.

While this wasn't the normal way a non-profit goes about forming its board of directors, the process worked. Later the board added Dr. David Hirsch, who also chaired the Medical Advisory Board. He primarily focused on convincing the Phoenix medical community, and pediatricians specifically, how crucial Ryan House would prove to be to their patients. Susan Levine and Debbie Shumway of Hospice of the Valley joined not long after. While Susan had initially told Holly that a children's hospice that also offered respite care was not something HOV felt compelled to build on its own, Susan had gone above and beyond to support the Cottors' efforts to make their dream a reality since the day Holly first came to see her. Not only did she provide meeting space, HOV also gave Ryan House a $25,000 grant to help hire its first Executive Director. Susan Levine said she'd commit another $25,000 for the Executive Director if the funds were needed. However, by the time the board found the right person to hire, the fundraising machine that was in motion covered that expense.

Passion from early board members and friends fueled countless, creative grassroots fundraisers: Former Indy car racer, Joey Truscelli, fostered a community march throughout Scottsdale's Grayhawk Community to announce a "Race for Ryan House" – the first fundraising event. The inaugural Paul Gavin Chait Memorial Golf Tournament and annual Memorial Event, followed soon after, as well as Family Harvest Picnic at the Arizona Biltmore. A number of third-party fundraisers not only raised needed funds, but helped introduce Ryan House to more caring hearts and friends: DC Ranch's Heartstrings Ball, Pioneer Ford's "Tricked Ponies" Mustang Car Show, Golf for Cause, The Little Gym's Holiday Auction, Avnet Jeans Day and many more! Age had no bounds either! From pre-K through upper school, Phoenix Country Day School students and staff benefited Ryan House with "Movie Night" through 2012, demonstrating their belief in being a private school with a public cause! On the other end of the spectrum, a senior citizen craft group at Westminster Village retirement community donated blankets. Each of these, and more, proved a labor of love and attested to the commitment for the future care of Ryan House.

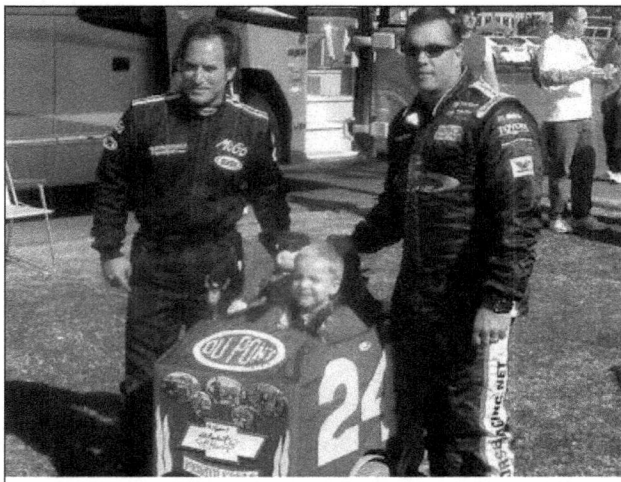

Joey T (left) with Ryan as Jeff Gordon and Fox Sports
NASCAR Commentator Jeff Hammond (right)

As the board came together and started meeting on a regular basis, further magic spread. Linda Hunt and St. Joseph's Medical Center finalized their gift of the land in the heart of Phoenix with no strings attached. Linda went out of her way to make it clear that Ryan House was not an extension of her hospital, but a completely independent entity that would just happen to be built down the street. But she didn't stop there. Between the time her board gave Ryan House its land on a sixty year, one dollar a year lease, and the day construction finally began, she battled with the city to make the house possible on the proposed site. City ordinances would not allow the house to be built as close to the street as the plans required. Linda went to city hall and asked that the street be made the private property of St. Joseph's. The city eventually agreed, only to then inform her that the street did not meet city codes. St. Joseph's had to bring the street, and its utilities underneath, up to date at a cost of hundreds of thousands of dollars. This was but the first of many battles Linda and others fought with city hall for Ryan House. She and Judy Schubert plus other board members called in every favor they possibly could to cut through miles of red tape. In the end they succeeded. It was pure magic, which, again, is defined as hard work fueled by tireless passion.

The house itself began to take shape as architectural plans, conceived by Orcutt Winslow Partnership, went through a series of revisions until the board settled on a final design. They now had something to show people as the fundraising kicked into gear. And fundraising was at the heart of the mission of the board of directors. Time after time Judy Schubert stood and lectured them: "If the money doesn't come in, we will not have a house!" Board members stepped up with donations of their own. One member became the house's single, largest donor with gifts totaling $350,000.

The Arizona Republic, Phoenix's largest daily newspaper, ran their first feature about the Cotters and Ryan House. Holly opened the paper and found a photograph of herself and Ryan on the first page of the Valley & State section. After the story ran, donations picked up. A women's poker group in nearby Peoria read the story and donated their weekly pot of $35. A prison inmate heard about Ryan House and started sending in eight dollars each month just to help the kids.

Grants also started to be awarded. St. Luke's Health Initiatives gave the first grant of $35,000. The board used the money to hire their first business consultant, Nancy Hook. Nancy worked closely with Jonathan to complete and formalize the business plan that Holly and Rachel Osterele had started in July, 2004. Over the next few years, grants from area businesses and foundations rolled in, including a $650,000 grant from the Virginia G. Piper Charitable Trust and a half million dollar grant from the Gila River Indian Community. School children rallied behind building Ryan House, with area schools such as Phoenix Country Day organizing Movie Night fundraisers for Ryan House where families made donations in lieu of a babysitter fee for the night. Other Arizona students donated money and gift cards for the house rather than receiving birthday gifts.

On top of all the grants and fundraising efforts, The Board of Visitors set their goal at one million dollars for Ryan House through the Care Card program. Formalizing the goal meant this was more than a one or two year commitment. Up until this time, the Care Card had raised less than $200,000 a year for their target charities. The BOV executive committee figured it would take at least six years to reach their million dollar goal. Although everyone expected Ryan House to be built in less time than that, the committee still went forward with it. Knowing the house's services were to be free of charge to all families that needed them, fundraising would always be a part of its mission. After The Board of Visitors stepped up with their million dollar plan in the fall of 2008, the Ryan House board officially renamed the House: "The Board of Visitors Ryan House."

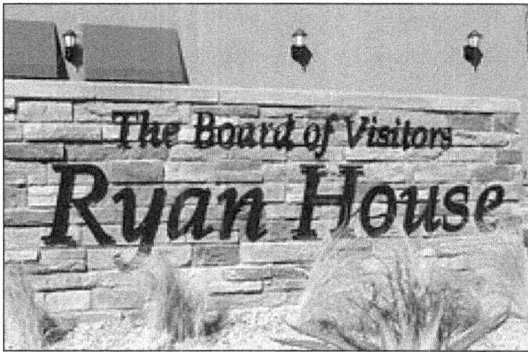

All of this took place over the course of the six years it took for Ryan House to go from an idea to an actual structure open for business. Excitement for the project spread through the community as the board worked diligently to get the word out about what Ryan House would do, as well as showcasing the children and families it would serve.

However, before the word could go out, the board had to clarify both its mission and the message. Early on, the message was very Helen House centered. Holly and Jonathan went around talking about their experiences there, while Jonathan repeatedly showed the Helen House video he'd first shown to the small group gathered in Judy Schubert's living room. Several of the founding board members traveled to England to see Helen House firsthand.

However, once Ryan House had its own name, location, and building plans, the message had to go far beyond comparisons to a children's hospice in England. The community needed to understand why another place dedicated to sick children was so necessary in Phoenix and what set this place apart from the Ronald McDonald House. The latter came up often then and it still does today.

Finding a way to clearly and effectively communicate the Ryan House message became Jon Ford's personal mission once he became part of the board of directors. Jon came on board with twenty years of experience in marketing and advertising. He'd worked with major brand names like Frito Lay, Tropicana and General Motors. That he even knew about Ryan House was just one more magical moment. Jon and his family lived in the Cottors' neighborhood and right next door to the neighborhood park. Many families who used the park ended up dropping by the Ford's house since they were the closest water source. One afternoon Jon noticed a new family playing in the park, a mom and dad with two young sons. But this family was a little different. The smallest boy could not play on the equipment by himself. He was also confined to a wheelchair. Jon went out and introduced himself. That's when his friendship with Jonathan and Holly began. Jon's two children were close in age to Ethan and Ryan, and the two families hit it off. Informal talks in the park got around to what each man did for a living, which led to Jonathan calling Jon one afternoon and inviting him to dinner. During dinner, Jonathan explained the vision for Ryan House and asked Jon to come on board. Of course he said yes.

Unlike other members of the board, Jon did not have any connections to the larger community. He'd only lived in Phoenix for a few years after moving there from Chicago. Nor did he have a fundraising background. But Jon had three things that Ryan House needed to get off the ground. First, he knew marketing and advertising. From the start he talked about the need for the house to create a brand identity which would make their mission clear and simple to understand. Selling the house to the community as a whole was crucial. Jon preached to the board that they needed to do more than raise funds to build the house. They needed to have the community own Ryan House to such a degree that the community would never let it die. People will write checks to good causes without fully buying into them. Jon wanted them to do more than reach Phoenix's wallets. He wanted the city to own this cause, to make it their own.

Second, Jon understood the fact that children with life threatening conditions are first and foremost children. As he developed a relationship with Ryan, he saw a little boy who refused to be defined by his condition. Jon wanted to make sure the community understood that none of these children should be labeled by their conditions, either. Once you label someone, they become a thing and not a person. In all of his marketing plans for the House, Jon wanted to make sure that the children Ryan House would serve remained children. The children's hospice model from England worked because families and children could go there and feel normal. Kids are kids, not kids with SMA or any other condition. They are just children. Ryan House had to do the same, and that applied not only within Ryan House, but in its message to the community as well.

Finally, through his relationship with the Cottor family, Jon knew this project was not only for children, but for families, too. Most studies find that a startling percentage of families with children who have life threatening conditions end up in divorce. The strain of continually providing the same level of care a newborn demands year after year eventually takes its toll. Yes, Ryan House was being designed for children, but Jon talked constantly of how those children cannot be separated from the lives of their families as a whole. He knew from experience that families function better when everyone gets a full night's sleep from time to time.

Because of his commitment to the sanctity of the family, Jon knew family preservation was a key part of the mission, even if no one ever put it into words. That was why he agreed to serve when he was invited to join the board. He looked beyond the house and focused on the families who desperately needed it.

Through interviews with the other board members, as well as talking with families like the Cottors, Jon set out to clearly define the brand personality of Ryan House. He found that three core mission points came up over and over again. First, they needed to provide essential care for the families and children. Second, everyone involved in the project did so because they wanted to help these children live their lives to the fullest. Finally, the organization was dedicated to providing community support for these families.

As the board refined these three core values, Jon created talking points and key messaging statements for the board to use when presenting Ryan House to the community. Within these talking points was a set of do's and don'ts. In the beginning, Holly talked about "hospice" and "palliative care." While both accurately describe the house's mission, neither really communicated to people outside the hospice and palliative care world. Jon replaced "hospice" with "end-of-life care," and "palliative care" with "special care to help children live life to the fullest." He also made sure every talking point emphasized "respite care for families." Everyone who spoke in public also worked hard not to paint a picture of sick and dying children in desperate need of help. Instead, they spoke of the children who would use Ryan House for what they are: children who deserve the best life possible.

While Jon worked on branding, Jonathan and Holly organized the first Ryan House open house for families. The house itself was still nothing more than a set of plans and a dirt lot, but that didn't matter. The Cottors put up a tent in a nearby park, ordered a six foot long party sub from a local sandwich shop, and invited all the families they knew who had children with life threatening conditions. It was the first of a long string of regular family events that continue on today. Their reason for holding the open house, then and now, is simple. Even if the Phoenix business and medical communities buy into Ryan House and even if magic strikes and money rolls in and the stars align to make the dream a reality, none of it matters if the families for whom the house was planned do not see it as their own. But once this community buys into it, not only will the house be built, it will remain a vital part of the community for as long as children are diagnosed with life threatening conditions.

Mikaela

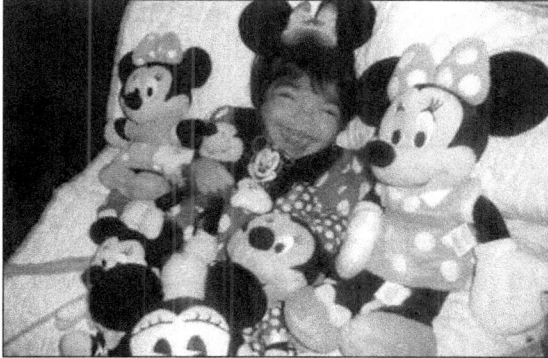

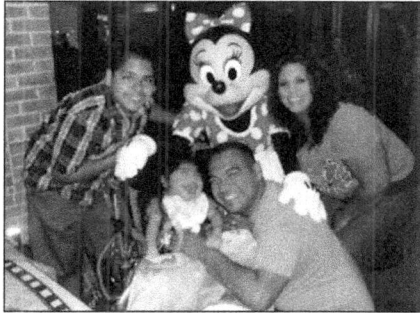

Mikaela was a fighter from the day she was born. She had to be. Before she was even born her doctors discovered problems with both her heart and lungs. "Your child probably won't survive. You should seriously consider terminating the pregnancy," her mother, Melody, was told. But Melody wouldn't hear of it. For six years she prayed for a daughter. If the baby growing inside her with defective heart and lungs was the child God chose to give her, Melody would love her and fight for her and do everything she could to give her the best life possible. "No," she told the doctors, "I'm going to care for my little girl no matter how sick she may be."

As Melody came closer to term, her doctors tried to prepare her for what she should expect when her child was born. "She'll come out blue from the lack of oxygen. And there's a chance..." Melody didn't have to hear the rest. She knew there was a chance her little girl might not survive birth.

"I think you will be surprised," Melody replied.

When Mikaela was born, she came out pink and crying like any other baby. Melody held her in her arms and wept. "You really are a miracle child," she whispered.

But Melody's time with Mikaela was cut short as the medical team rushed her off to the cardiac ICU. Mikaela was born with heart disease, chronic lung disease, severe scoliosis and cerebral palsy. Melody and her husband were told the baby would not survive six months. Six days later the prediction appeared to be overly optimistic as Mikaela coded for the first time. It happened suddenly. Melody was sitting in the ICU unit, rocking Mikaela in her arms, when suddenly she stopped breathing. A team of doctors and nurses rushed in and worked frantically. They revived her but the next four days were touch and go as they kept her on life support. Mikaela fought just as hard for her life.

She kept fighting throughout her first year, all of which but a few weeks were spent in St. Joseph's Hospital. Melody managed to bring her home for a couple of weeks, but Mikaela soon developed an infection and ended up back in the hospital. Throughout her hospital stays in 2008 and 2009, Melody noticed a large sign in front of a construction near the hospital. "The future home of Ryan House," it read. She'd heard of the place on the news and on the Care Card billboards around town over the past few years, but she never thought about it as something for her and her family.

During a hospital stay in early 2010 the empty lot had become a very active construction site. Melody decided to walk over and check it out for herself. The house was close to completion, but it was still a construction area. She returned a second time shortly before the House's grand opening. Pam Roman, the Team Leader, greeted her at the door. Melody told her all about Mikaela and the doctors' grim prognosis. "Your daughter is exactly the kind of child we're building this place for," Pam told her with a smile.

Melody was a little unsure what that meant. "How so?" she asked.

Pam explained the mission of Ryan House and how it would provide a place for respite for parents. "We're going to open in a couple of weeks, so you dropped by at a really good time," Pam said. "We can even schedule a respite stay for you now for any time in the next few months. Since we haven't opened yet, we have a lot of open slots."

The more Pam talked about respite, the more interested Melody became. The past year had pushed her to her limits. Every day she got up early and went to work. As soon as she got off at three in the afternoon, she rushed to the hospital to stay by Mikaela's side. At midnight she finally went home, and then got up early the next morning to do it all over again. Her husband spent as much time as he could at the hospital as well, but the two of them hardly had any time for each other or for their older son. They were only a little over a year in, and already she knew she was closing in on her breaking point.

"Would you like the tour?" Pam asked.

"I guess so," Melody said, still a little uncertain about the place. Up until this point in her short life, Mikaela had spent so much time in hospitals that they were nearly the only home she'd known. Walking through Ryan House, Melody was struck by how non-hospital it appeared. "This place looks like Disneyland for a special needs child," Melody said.

"That's the idea," Pam replied.

After the tour, Melody booked a stay for Mikaela at Ryan House for July, which was just four months away. Making the reservation was a bit of an act of faith after how Mikaela's first year had gone. But life with Mikaela had been a journey of faith since before she was born. She'd already beaten the odds by living past her first birthday. Melody felt confident she would indeed get to stay at Ryan House that summer.

Melody brought Mikaela home from the hospital for good later that spring. However, she remained a very sick little girl. The doctors had to insert a trach for her to breathe with the aid of a ventilator because of the problems with her lungs. Having a ventilator in their home also meant regular deliveries of bottles of oxygen. Someone always had to keep a close eye on Mikaela because the trach had to be suctioned out on a regular basis to remain clear. Mikaela was unable to eat on her own, which meant she had to have a G-tube inserted.

Once Mikaela came home, the family settled into an exhausting routine. State medical coverage for special needs children pro-vided a day nurse who stayed with Mikaela while Melody and her husband went to work. After work, Melody's second job started. From the moment she got home from work a little after three in the afternoon, Mikaela's care consumed all of her time. Mikaela liked spending time with her mother so much that she slept during the day while Melody was at work then stayed awake all through the night. Melody managed to catch a little sleep here and there, but nothing close to the level she needed to function normally.

When July rolled around, Melody and her husband were eager for a break. They filled their Suburban with Mikaela's special chair, a custom stroller, four three and a half feet long oxygen bottles, suc-tion machine, ventilator, diapers, clothes, toys and all her medica-tion and headed toward downtown Phoenix from her home an hour away in Surprise, Arizona. It took Melody three trips to carry every-thing from the car into Mikaela's Ryan House room, and nearly an hour to arrange everything exactly the way she wanted it. "I don't mean to be so picky," she explained to the caregiver who was help-ing her, "but I want it to feel as much like home as possible."

"Take all the time you need," was the reply.

Once Mikaela was settled into her room, Melody returned to the reception area to finish the paperwork. When she returned to the room a short while later, Mikaela was not there. Melody looked around the halls and finally found her in the sensory room with Gabrielle, one of the house volunteers. She stood back and watched. Gabrielle cradled Mikaela in her arms and talked to her like she was a typical child, not a sick little girl. She pointed and laughed and giggled. Mikaela beamed with a huge smile as the lights danced around her. Melody turned and hurried out, fighting back tears. In all the months in the hospital, Melody had never witnessed anyone speak to Mikaela like that. It felt like everyone always spoke down to her, like she was fragile or already broken. Gabrielle spoke to her like she was her own child. Any reservations Melody had about leaving her little girl evaporated. She knew she was in good hands.

When Melody and her husband returned a week later after a vacation for just the two of them, she was surprised to find Mikaela was not ready to leave. Her big smile that she always wore went away, replaced by an unmistakable frown. "Don't worry, baby, we'll come back. Don't worry. You'll get to come back here."

After that, Melody arranged regular stays for Mikaela. Not all of them were planned well in advance. At one point, Melody knew she'd reached her breaking point. The lack of sleep coupled with having no time for anything but caring for her little girl, along with going back and forth between hospital stays had worn her down. She called Ryan House and spoke with Pam. "Help," she said, "I have to have a break. Do you have room for Mikaela?"

"When would you like for her to come?"

"Now," came the desperate reply.

"We can do that," Pam said.

Melody loaded up the Suburban and moved Mikaela in for a few days. This time she didn't go away on vacation. She went home and slept.

Even with the respite breaks, the stress of caring for such a sick little girl and the lack of time for one another led to the dissolution of Melody and her husband's marriage. They remained on good terms for the sake of their children but the marriage could not survive all the two of them had gone through. They are not alone. Close to ninety percent of marriages in families with a special needs child end up in divorce. Ultimately, Melody also had to quit her job to care for Mikaela full time. More close calls came when she did not know if her little girl would live or die. Each time Mikaela fought through it. Doctors repeatedly came and told Melody that she was going to have to make a difficult decision, and every time Mikaela rallied and ended up going home. She continually beat the odds. Melody prayed she always would.

Make a Wish threw a Disney princess party for Mikaela at the Phoenix Children's Museum. Jenni Rogers and several of the other Ryan House Care Team members attended. A limo came to the house and picked up Mikaela and Melody. When they arrived at the Museum, they were greeted by Snow White, Belle and Sleeping Beauty. A stylist came and did Mikaela's hair and nails. Melody watched Mikaela enjoy the moment. Her little girl truly was a princess.

In the last year of her life, Mikaela stayed out of the hospital completely. She even got to spend her last Christmas at home with her mom and dad. Every other Christmas had been spent in a hospital room, but they finally got to enjoy the holidays together. Even though they were divorced, Melody and Mikaela's father spent the entire day together with their children. Mikaela's daily care still wore Melody down but Mikaela seemed to be growing stronger. The next spring they took Mikaela to Disneyland. She loved "It's a Small World" and the "Pirates of the Caribbean" rides most of all. Mickey Mouse and Goofy and the other characters flocked to her. It was a special day.

However, by May, 2013, her health started to deteriorate. She developed infection after infection. Trips to the doctor's office and new medications always seemed to clear them up, but the frequency of the infections was disconcerting. In June she became sick once more. Melody hoped Mikaela had come down with the same bug that everyone seemed to have, but this was more than a summer cold. Mikaela labored with each breath.

Melody rushed her to Phoenix Children's Hospital on a Monday. Doctors found she had pneumonia and a urinary tract infection. The two had left her very dehydrated. Once again, the medical team talked to Melody and Mikaela's father about the hard choices they would have to soon make. "We aren't ready to do that," Melody replied. On Tuesday her fever spiked. Her doctors put her on three new heart medications to keep her alive. Mikaela had always been a fighter, but by Wednesday she was too tired to fight. Melody kissed her little girl on the forehead and whispered in her ear, "It's okay, baby. You've fought so hard. You can go run and play in heaven now."

When she was born the doctors said Mikaela would not live six months. She beat that estimate by four years. Like any little girl, she had lots of favorite things. She loved Disney princesses and Mickey Mouse. And she had a favorite place where she loved to go and stay. That place was Ryan House. When she came through the door she always broke out into a giant grin. She had the same effect on everyone there who cared for her. That's what makes Ryan House such a special place.

Chapter Nine

Game Changer

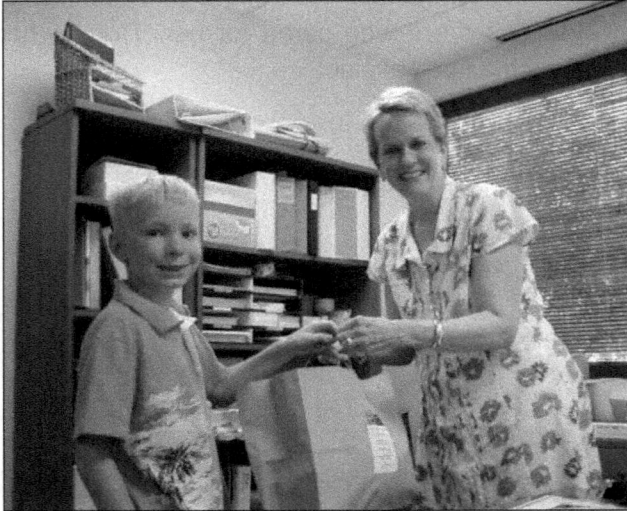

Nancy Martin, Ryan House's first Executive Director,
receiving birthday gift donations from Ethan

NANCY MARTIN DECIDED TO DROP by to see an old friend before she headed back to Kentucky. Although a native of Tucson and a longtime resident of Phoenix, Nancy and her husband had lived all across the country over the previous thirteen years. Her husband had recently retired, and Nancy planned to retire the following year after she finished her work with a Kentucky non-profit organization. After retirement, they planned on moving back to the warmth and sunshine of Arizona. But on this day she was simply back visiting family and friends. That's why she decided to drop in on Judy Schubert. The two had been friends for thirty-five years and had worked together on the Ronald McDonald House before Nancy moved away.

The two friends started catching up, as friends will do. "Are you still with that group in Alabama?" Judy asked.

"We're in Kentucky now," Nancy replied. "Bill's already retired and he's anxious for me to do the same. I told him to give me one more year then I will hang it up."

"And then what?" Judy asked.

"And then we come back here. I don't think I can handle another winter back east. Besides, I'm an Arizona girl. I'm ready to come home."

"How would you feel about coming back a little sooner?" Judy asked with a twinkle in her eye.

"Why? What are you up to?"

Judy then proceeded to fill Nancy in on her work with Ryan House. "We hope to open in 2008 or 2009. But to get there we need to hire a really good executive director who knows this community, has experience helping a non-profit get off the ground, and who can raise a lot of money." Judy then sat back and smiled.

"Judy," Nancy replied, "I'm a year from retirement."

"I was hoping I could talk you into putting it off for a little while," Judy said.

"I don't know...? I guess I could consider it, but I doubt if Bill will go along with it."

"Well, you never know. Give it some thought, talk to him about it and get back with me."

A few weeks later Nancy was back in Phoenix for a job interview she never expected. She'd done a quick study on the board's progress to this point and had also read *A House Called Helen*. Her experience with non-profits all over the country told her that actually moving from idea to reality was far more difficult than anyone probably imagined. The prospect of raising seven million dollars made her feel more than a little ill. After all, she knew that in spite of its size, Phoenix was really a small community. Every group went to the same individuals and corporations for money for their worthy causes. There was only so much cash to go around. Raising enough to both build the house and create an endowment for its long term sustainability was not going to be easy. However, she knew Judy Schubert and a few other board members quite well. *If they think it can be done, then it probably can*, she told herself.

The board agreed that she was the one who could help make it happen and offered her the job.

A week later as a board meeting ended, Judy Schubert and Susan Levine walked out the door together. "So what are your plans for the rest of the week?" Susan asked, making conversation.

"I need to start hunting for a place to get benefits for our soon to be one employee. Have any ideas where I should start?"

"Start with us."

"What?"

"Why don't I fold her into Hospice of the Valley to start? We have the benefit structure in place. We can just sort of adopt her for a little while until Ryan House is completely set up."

Judy let out a relieved sigh. "That's one headache solved. Now I just need to find an office space to rent and everything will be in place for Nancy to hit the ground running when she comes next month."

"I think I can find a corner for her in our building across the street from here. We need all the money we can find to get this house up and running without wasting any on rent," Susan said.

A month later Nancy arrived and got to work. She started plotting out all the things Ryan House needed to operate both now and into the future. By her second week of driving up to the HOV offices, a thought hit her. *Hospice of the Valley is one of the largest, most respected non-profit hospices in the country. They're already doing a lot of what we plan to do, and they already have knowledge and experience operating hospice units and care teams along with a volunteer training program. They also have many of the other administrative functions. I'm going to have to start from scratch. And they have space for all these people and departments and more space planned to accommodate future growth. What if...?* She called Judy Schubert. "Judy. I have an idea. It's something completely different from what we've talked about so far, but I think it just might make our work and the work of those who come after us a whole lot easier."

"I'm game," Judy replied. After listening to Nancy's idea, Judy said, "I've been thinking about the need for the very same thing. Let's put something together and talk to Susan."

A few days later, Nancy and Judy sat down in Susan's office. "Susan, we have an idea we would like for you to consider." Nancy handed Susan a draft of a proposal they had cranked out over the weekend while staying in Judy's guesthouse. "As we started working on the Ryan House organization and charting out the infrastructure we're going to need long term, it hit us. With all of the departments and personnel we need to create for what is, essentially, a rather small operation in terms of the number of children and families with whom we will work at any one time, well, it just doesn't make sense for us to try to go it alone. I talked to the director of George Mark Children's House in California and they found this out the hard way. They ended up with a much larger support staff than anyone ever anticipated. They didn't build enough space for everyone they needed and they sure didn't budget for them. So what would you think about us partnering with you and Hospice of the Valley in the areas where we naturally overlap?"

"What do you mean?"

Judy spoke up. "Take nursing care, for example. We're going to have to have enough nurses available for a full house. But what about the days when we only have one or two rooms filled? We're going to have all that extra staff that we still need to pay when there's nothing for them to do. But we can't hire people to only work on an as needed basis. That isn't fair to us or them. But if we partner with you, perhaps our nursing staff could flex into your system for work on days that Ryan House may not need them and we can share their salary costs? When I think of long term sustainability, I know we're going to have to find ways like this to keep our expenses under control."

Judy shared more, "I'm really worried about how much money we're going to need to raise each year to keep the doors open. I also talked to the director of George Mark Children's House last week. She told me their annual budget is much larger than it should be because they are completely on their own. Even though they are small in terms of the number of families they serve at any one time, just like we will be, they still have to staff for all the varied needs of the kids they have. I don't think that model can work long term. We have to get our costs down to a sustainable level and I think this partnership is a way to do that."

"I think this makes a lot of sense. Let me read through your proposal and take it to my board. I will get back with you," Susan replied.

Not long after this meeting, the board sent Nancy to England to tour the children's hospices there, beginning with Helen House. Several board members had already made the trip and all agreed the best way to understand exactly what they wanted to do was to familiarize themselves with the care models throughout the UK that were working so well.

Nancy's experience with Helen House was a little different than that of the Cottors or Linda Hunt who had also visited. Sister Frances, who actually started Helen House as a result of caring for a little girl named Helen Worswick, greeted Nancy in a very polite, yet rather distant way. "I'm the executive director of a place called Ryan House in Arizona. We hope to open our house in two years if everything comes together the way we expect," Nancy said.

"Oh," Sister Frances replied in a flat tone. She then proceeded to show Nancy around in a very direct, matter of fact, *let's get this over with quickly* sort of way. Nancy tried to engage her in conversation, asking about the day-to-day operations and how they handled issues which Nancy had encountered already. Sister Frances's answers were always clipped and unenthusiastic.

Finally, Nancy asked, "So what advice can you give that would be most helpful in starting a house like this?"

"I don't think it can be done," was the response.

Nancy looked at her with surprise.

"No offense to you or your organization," Sister Frances continued, "I'm sure they're all lovely people with very good intentions, but I have had scores of lovely people with good intentions from the States come over here and tour our home and tell me how they are going to build something just like it in their neighborhood, and none of them have ever succeeded. Honestly, I don't think it ever can be done on your side of the pond."

Nancy pushed further. "W...why do you think that is?"

"In a word, money. Replicating what we have done here is just too expensive in your American system. Every group runs into the same problem. A place like this is expensive to build. It is expensive to run. And it is expensive to keep in operation year after year after year. Frankly, I don't think it can be done in your country, no offense to you personally."

"I, uh, I don't know what to say," Nancy said.

"My dear, I really don't mean to discourage you and I apologize if I seem a little abrupt. I don't mean to come across that way. I am just being honest with you since you asked for my advice. So many people have come over and asked me the same question, all of them just as sincere and well intentioned as you are today. Yet all of them have ended up defeated. I simply don't want to fill you with false hope. Replicating what we have here may not be possible in America."

"We will be the first," Nancy said.

"I hope you are," Sister Frances replied.

After her return from England, Nancy traveled to San Leandro, California to visit George Mark Children's House. Susan Levine joined her on that trip. After touring the House, Nancy and Susan sat down with the George Mark executive director and asked, "What do we need to know to make our house a success?"

Her George Mark counterpart didn't even pause before answering. "I wish we'd partnered with a local hospital or hospice. Operating any kind of medical facility in California, or anywhere, is very regulated and expensive. We could save so much in terms of both time and money if we hadn't completely reinvented the wheel here and found a partner."

Susan and Nancy exchanged a knowing look. This confirmed the conversations they'd already had about partnering together. "Why didn't you?" Susan asked.

"Independence. When George Mark began, we had the good fortune of financial freedom thanks to the significant generosity of our founder, Kathy Hull. We built our vision without having to worry about money. But in hindsight, we now wish we had done more to build support in the community. We're playing catch up now, but it's hard. If we could do it all over again, we would start reaching out to the community before we turned over the first shovel full of dirt. A place like this faces a real uphill climb if the community doesn't buy into it completely."

"That's what we're doing in Phoenix," Nancy said. "It's been that way from the start."

"Don't stop!"

"Don't worry. We won't," Nancy said with a smile.

Not long after the trip to San Leandro, Nancy joined Judy for a meeting in Susan's office. Debbie Shumway, HOV's then associate executive director joined them. When the conversation turned to the possible partnership between Hospice of the Valley and Ryan House, Susan had a surprise prepared. "This is going to sound crazy but what if we put a second floor on Ryan House that could be a palliative care unit for adults?"

"Okay...what?" Judy said, more than a little confused.

"Instead of a one story structure with eight rooms and four family suites, what if we make it a two story structure with twelve rooms upstairs. Upstairs would be ours, and the downstairs would be yours."

"I think that sounds like a great idea," Judy said. She and other board members had already started thinking about the long-term needs of the children of Ryan House who age out and could not stay at the House any longer. Helen House met this need by creating Douglas House for young adults with life limiting conditions. Judy immediately thought of Douglas House. To her, Susan's suggestion sounded like a godsend. "Before I can say okay, I need to talk to Linda Hunt. She and St. Joe's gave us the land. Well, I mean they leased it to us for a dollar a year for sixty years. I need to make sure having two facilities in one building on the site is okay with her. If it is, I will take this to our board."

Nancy nodded in agreement. "I like your idea," she said. "I like it a lot."

The next time Judy met with Susan, the "second floor" had evolved even more. "Why don't we at HOV just build the whole thing?" Susan said.

Once Judy picked herself up off the floor, she replied, "Are you serious!?"

"Of course. I talked it over with my board, and we think it only makes sense. We have the money to do it, and, as a non-profit organization, we want to pour our resources back into the community. I believe very strongly in the mission of Ryan House. If I didn't, I wouldn't be on the board. I want to see this house built and succeed as badly as anyone else."

"Oh my gosh, Susan, I don't know what to say."

Susan smiled. "I'm excited, too. We'll pay the construction costs. Ryan House will cover the costs to furnish it and equip it and all of that."

"Of course," Judy said.

"Now, to make this work, we need to have Ryan House do three things. First, before construction begins, you need to have three years of operating expenses in the bank. That will ease the team from the worry of operating month-to-month on a shoe-string budget."

Judy nodded. "That makes sense. We've raised close to two and a half million so far." She broke out in a grin, "Which means we can now roll most of that over into our operations budget since we don't have to build a house!"

The two of them laughed. "That's wonderful, isn't it?" Susan said. "The second request from my board is that you start an endowment to help fund the operations of the house long term."

"I've already been thinking about how we need to do that," Judy replied.

"And the final thing is, you will pay all the operating costs for the first floor. That will keep your board connected and they will have skin-in-the-game. Your board needs to recognize that they need to continue to work hard to raise the annual operating expenses each and every year."

"That all sounds very doable." Judy let out a long sigh as if a weight had been lifted off her shoulders. "I can't wait to tell our board about this."

"Do you think all of them will go for this? I know some of them really want to remain completely independent," Susan said.

"I think they will go for it as long as Jonathan does."

"Will he?" Susan asked.

"Let's go talk to him," Judy said.

Susan and Judy asked Jonathan to meet without telling him exactly what the two of them had in mind. As the three sat down, Susan began. "Jonathan, when Holly first came to me with the idea to build Ryan House, honesty, I was skeptical that you all could pull it off. But, as we've been on this journey together, I have become a real believer. At this point, I want to do everything I can to make sure your dream becomes a reality."

"I can't tell you how much that means to us," Jonathan said.

"So I have an idea that might make that reality come sooner rather than later." Susan smiled and glanced over at Judy. "What if Hospice of the Valley builds Ryan House?" Susan said.

Jonathan sat back in his chair, speechless. *I think she just handed us a $6.5 million check*, he thought. He paused for a very long time, then gathered himself and said, "Meaning what exactly?"

"Meaning we build the house," Susan replied.

He looked over at Judy. "Is she serious?"

Judy broke out in a huge grin. "Yes, she is," she said.

Susan continued, "You all have raised over $2.5 million so far. We want you to keep it and shift the funds you've raised to your operational fund to assure there is plenty of money when the house opens."

"This is fantastic!" Jonathan said, hardly able to believe what he was hearing. Then reality sat in. *What's the catch?* he wondered.

"Judy and I have been talking about ways to assure the long-term sustainability of Ryan House. What we would like to do to help manage costs, is create a twelve bedroom palliative care unit on a second floor of Ryan House," explained Susan.

And there it is. His enthusiasm drained. "Are you suggesting that this becomes a twenty bedroom facility? This is a house. We call it Ryan *House* for a reason. It's supposed to feel like a second home for these families, not another medical facility."

"No, no, no, Jonathan," Susan replied. "I am not suggesting we change any of that. What Judy and I have discussed is creating something entirely new, with two separate organizations co-existing on the same footprint but operating separately. We at HOV know how to run adult hospice homes. We have seventeen of them around the Valley. This would be our eighteenth. By doing this, we can leverage building costs and share some day-to-day costs to reduce Ryan House's overall expenses."

Judy added, "And Jonathan, with the second floor in place, the possibility of someday continuing the care for these children who do live beyond eighteen could be already in place. Just like Helen House did with Douglas House."

"I love that vision!" Jonathan grinned.

"Let's not get ahead of ourselves. Right now we still have lots and lots of work to do to make Ryan House for kids sustainable long into the future. But, it does set things up really well for future growth," Susan said.

Jonathan had lots of questions and Susan and Judy took the time to bring him up to speed on their conversations to date. By the time they finished, his reservations were gone. "I say we do it. This is a huge win for Ryan House," he said to Judy.

Tears welled up in her eyes. "Yes it is," she said. "Yes it is."

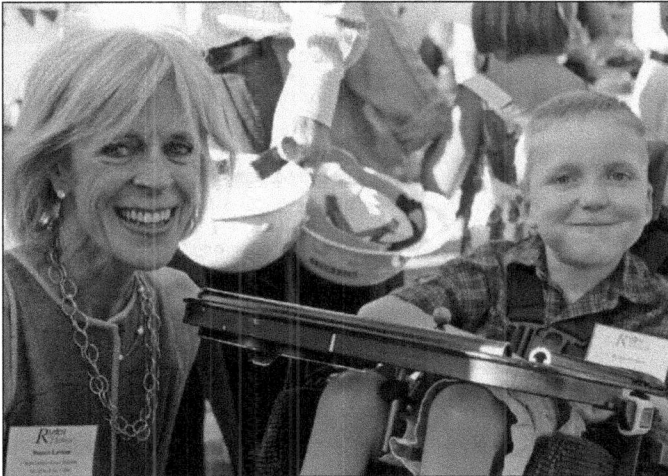

Susan Levine and Ryan during groundbreaking ceremony

Chapter Ten

Breaking Ground

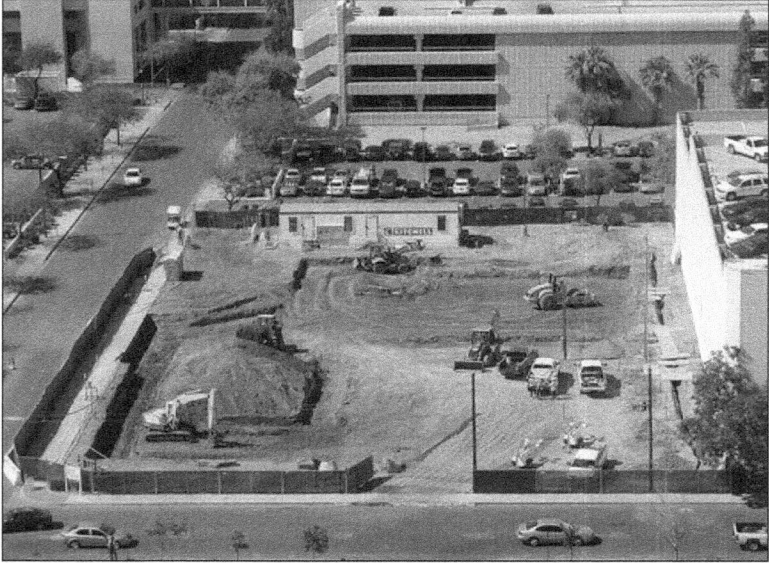

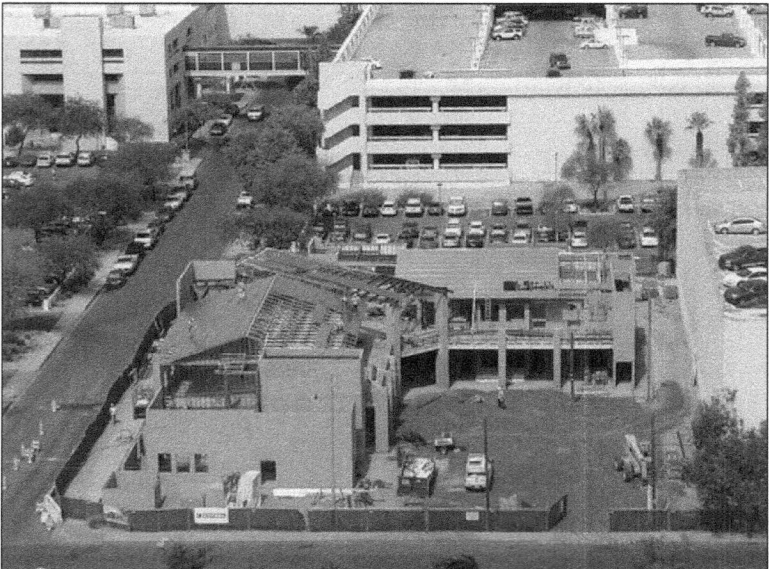

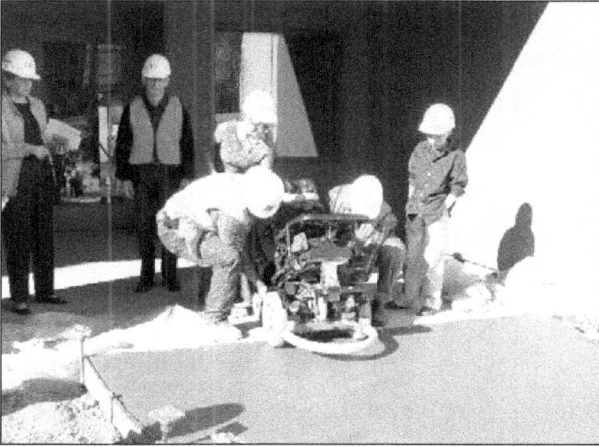

Lifting Ryan's wheelchair to mark Ryan's and Ethan's
hand prints on the outdoor patio of Ryan House

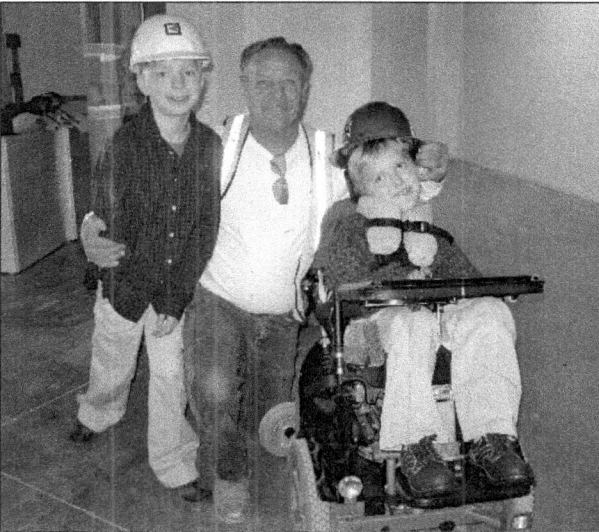

Ethan and Ryan with the Kitchell foreman

NOT EVERY MEMBER OF THE Ryan House board of directors jumped at the
chance to accept Susan Levine's offer to build the house as part of a partnership between the two organizations. "Won't making it a part of Hospice of the
Valley pretty much destroy all the effort we put into trying to convince people

that this isn't a hospice, at least, not what most people traditionally think of as a hospice," the objection came.

"And how do we know we won't end up being swallowed up by HOV?" came another. "We will cease to be what we set out to become. Then what will we have if the house doesn't do what we envisioned from the beginning?"

"We won't let that happen," Judy Schubert reassured everyone. "The proposed agreement makes that very clear. Our mission will not change and HOV is not going to tell us how to do our stuff. We will still be an independent board that will have the final say in what we do. No one is going to make those decisions for us. And we're still going to pay our own way, starting with equipping and furnishing our half of the building. That's all up to us, just as we've planned all along."

"But you've put a second floor on the house. Now, instead of an eight bedroom house for children, you have a twenty room *facility* and there's no way we'll be able to create the culture that feels like home."

"Yes, there will be a second floor, but the two floors will not be one big facility," Judy countered. "We will be two completely separate entities who happen to share the same footprint. The first floor will not interact with the second and vice versa. Ryan House is the first floor. Period. And HOV has the second floor, but no more."

"How do we know HOV won't try to take over slowly over time?" someone asked.

Susan Levine spoke up. "HOV has absolutely no interest in doing that. Why would we? Listen, I believe in the mission of Ryan House as much as anyone in this room. That's why I made this offer and why I believe a partnership is the best way for Ryan House to succeed long term. Having one of our homes on the second floor means Ryan House can open sooner, not later, because we're going to build it now, while still retaining its independence. I think it's a win-win for both of us."

"Coming under HOV's umbrella helps us in another major way too," Jonathan added. "This partnership will allow us to operate under HOV's existing hospice license, something we just could not do as an independent entity.

While the majority of our services are respite and there still is no insurance reimbursement for that type of care, by operating under a hospice license we will be able to secure some insurance and Medicaid funds to support our end-of-life services. Every dollar helps." The board agreed.

"And don't forget this saves us so much time and money," Judy Shannon added. "We've been raising money for a few years now, and it has gone really well. We're at 2.5 million right now, which is incredible. But 2.5 is still quite a ways from 6.5 million. With this agreement in place, we can begin the construction phase which will also greatly help our fundraising efforts as the community can see our progress."

That ended the discussion. The board voted to move forward with finalizing the agreement. The board set up a sub-committee to work out the details. Attorneys for both Ryan House and HOV formalized the partnership agreement. While much of the final language was legalese, some very key aspects were robustly discussed and debated to assure the language was clear and appropriate for what both groups wanted. To operate under Hospice of the Valley's hospice license, it was important that all employees in the house were technically HOV employees since, ultimately, HOV was responsible for managing the license and the care of the families. However, the Ryan House board wanted to be sure that the community understood that HOV had not taken over the project entirely. After all, the Ryan House board would continue to raise money and pay for everything that happened on the first floor.

The language of the partnership agreement also made it clear that the senior staff of Ryan House, specifically the Executive Director who was responsible for the administration roles, and the Director of Inpatient Services, who would oversee the care team, both reported to the Ryan House board chair and Ryan House board. They would not report to HOV's board. This important clarification affects all decision-making as it related to day-to-day operations at Ryan House.

Kelly Mooney, one of Ryan House's board members and an attorney herself, along with Jonathan Cottor, spent many hours fine-tuning the final language of the documents along with the job descriptions for the senior Ryan

House roles. They also crafted an organizational chart to assure everything was synchronized. They, and everyone involved, wanted this unique relationship to be clear and hoped that it would become a model for other communities to emulate as they strived to build a Helen House type organization in their town. It was a great day when Judy Schubert, the then Board Chair of Ryan House, and Susan Levine, the Executive Director of Hospice of the Valley signed the agreement and made it official.

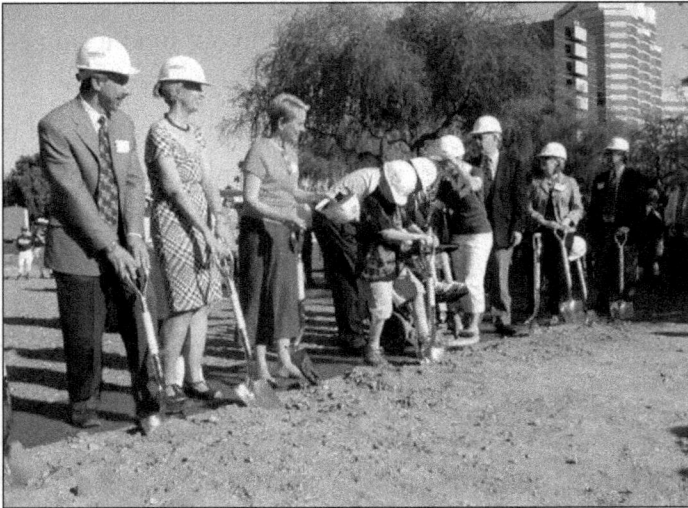

(From Left) Nabil AbouHaidar-Principal Architect, Kathleen Kassman-2007-2008 JLP President, Nancy Martin-1st Executive Director of Ryan House, and the Cottor Family during the Ceremonial Ground Breaking

The project now picked up speed like a train charging down the tracks. Architectural responsibility was now with Orcutt Winslow Partnership. Principal Architect Nabil Abou-Haidar, who had already drawn up several different designs, was hard at work making the final design of the two story building. Interior designer Suzanne Hanson, who had also partnered with Judy Schubert years earlier to bring the first Ronald McDonald House to Phoenix, had already started working on turning the space into a home-like environment. Another board member, Patty Taylor, spent time at George Mark Children's House, measuring and, with help from her own children armed with disposable cameras, photographing every inch as part of the design process.

George Mark's team continued to be very supportive throughout Ryan House's development, and was very willing and open about sharing their information and experiences. Kitchell Construction early on committed to waive their usual administrative fees to build Ryan House as had most of the subcontractors with whom they worked. The boards of Hospice of the Valley and Ryan House both agreed to keep all three on the project.

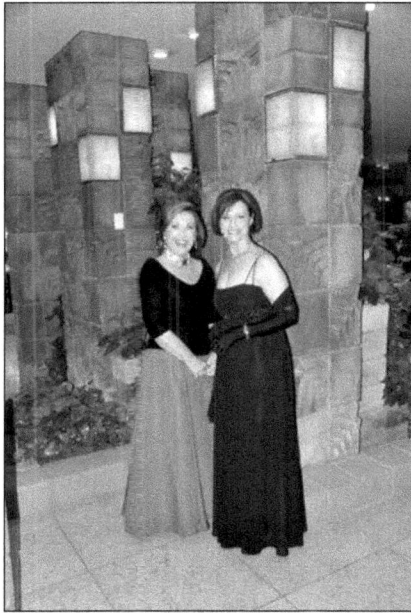

Jan Johnson and Judy Shannon at the White Christmas Event

With the pieces in place to start construction, fundraising became more intense, and, in some ways, easier. No longer were people asked to give on faith that Ryan House could be built. Bill and Judy Schubert graciously agreed to chair the formal capital committee. With their leadership, this amazing committee met frequently with the goal of raising $6.5 Million (later increased to $7.5 Million) to cover construction costs, fixtures and furnishings, and an initial nest egg of funds to cover the first few years of operating costs before the doors even opened.

Now Jan Johnson (who had been hired to coach the capital campaign) and the board could show potential donors the final drawings along with a realistic target opening date. Having HOV fully on board as a partner gave the project even greater credibility. Donations started coming in at a faster rate. Ryan House captured the community's imagination. School children began holding Ryan House fundraisers: movie nights, student council donations, and, eventually, sales of *One Raspberry*, a book written and donated by Gerda Weissmann Klein. The Run for Ryan House at DC Ranch, which began in 2004 with a 10K and 5K run, later added a Half Marathon and a One Mile Family Fun Run to raise money for the House. Eventually, it evolved into an annual event with more than 1,400 runners participating. More than funds, the Run for Ryan House created a great deal of awareness in the community as a whole.

In addition to the Run, in December, 2008, the board held its first White Christmas fundraiser at the prestigious Arizona Biltmore resort, which was attended by many of the most influential people in the Valley. Jan Johnson had been saving the idea for a White Christmas event for years, until she felt the perfect non-profit fit. Ryan House was once again at the right place at the right time. That event alone netted $101,000 its first year. The Arizona Biltmore also hosted regular Community Breakfasts, an integral part of fund-raising for many non-profits in the Phoenix area.

All together, these events, along with The Board of Visitors and Junior League of Phoenix Care Card and hundreds of spontaneous efforts by groups and individuals, proved so successful that Ryan House reached its $7 million goal by the time the House opened in March, 2010, two years after the agreement with HOV was finalized.

Phoenix mayor Phil Gordon declared April 23, 2008 "Ryan House Day" in the city as part of the formal groundbreaking ceremony. The ground was broken but full scale construction would not begin for several months. The board kept going back and forth on the overall layout of the building. Above all else, it had to look like a house, not a "facility." They finally settled upon a V design, where all of the bedrooms looked out onto a central courtyard and playground area. The great room, which provides a central living room, was placed at the center of the V. The kitchen was near the living room, which is where it needs to be in any well-designed house, while the special rooms for the children ran along one hall beyond the kitchen. Down the other end of the V was the central area for the Care Team, bathing room, family suites and sanctuary. At the time, no one anticipated the long hall that stretched from one end of the V to the other would become a race track for children in their power chairs, but ultimately that's what it became. It's part of what gives Ryan House its unique charm.

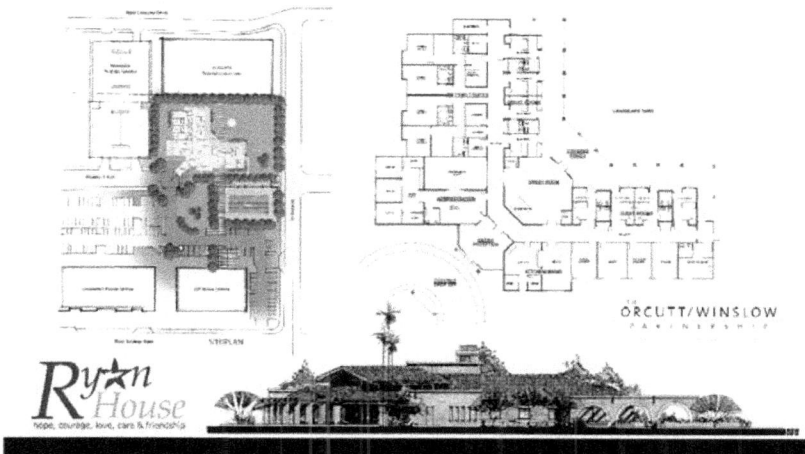

Ryan House site plan used during community presentations

After the groundbreaking, and before the actual construction began, the building's footprint was spray painted onto the lot at First and Merrell. Nancy took one group of potential donors after another there for a "tour". One group to whom she went to ask for a grant was The Thunderbirds, one of the leading philanthropic men's groups in the Phoenix area. A few days after her initial contact with the group, their leadership team met her at the building site which was still nothing more than a dirt lot with spray painted lines scattered about. They walked around, looking the site over carefully.

"What's this going to be?" one man asked, pointing to a jumble of lines in the center.

"Our playground. We are going to build it with playground equipment kids in wheelchairs can use," Nancy replied.

"That sounds expensive."

"I've talked to the people who come in and build it on site. They said it will probably cost around $150,000," Nancy said.

The men looked at one another and nodded. A few days later they called and said, "We're going to take care of your playground for you. We'll get a check to you by the end of the week."

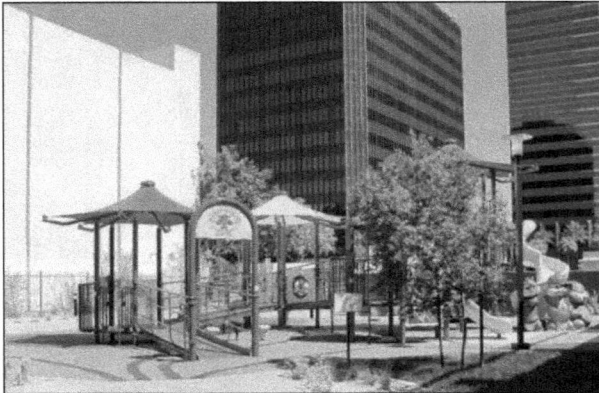

Ryan House's fully accessible playground thanks to the Thunderbirds!

Throughout construction, Nancy and members of the board continued working hard and reaching out to groups like The Thunderbirds. As word continued to get out throughout the community, some groups actually came to Ryan House asking what they could do to help. The manager of the Arizona Biltmore called Nancy one day. "Nancy, we're redecorating all our outdoor spaces, and we have a lot of outdoor furniture we can no longer use. Why don't you come over and take whatever you want?"

Another day, the owner of a high-end furniture store called. "I hear you're building a house," he said.

"We certainly are," Nancy replied.

"A house needs furniture, doesn't it?"

"Yes."

"We'd like to furnish it for you, the sofas and chairs, that sort of thing. Would that be okay?"

"Yes, I think it would be," Nancy said with a grin.

She had a very similar conversation with another man who called and asked a very open ended question, "What do you need?"

"Excuse me," Nancy replied.

"I heard about how you guys are building this Ryan House and I think it's a great idea. So what do you need?"

"Are you offering...?"

"Yeah, I just want to know what you need first."

"We could use televisions for the rooms," Nancy replied.

"How many do you need? And are flat screens okay?" This conversation was hardly unusual. Many suppliers stepped up and either donated or provided, at a substantial discount, many of the fixtures for the house. Individuals continued sending in donations as the board kept working hard to create ever more community awareness of Ryan House and its mission. To all those working twelve to fourteen hours a day trying to open Ryan House as soon as possible, every gift, no matter how small, was just as important as the six figure donations from area businesses and foundations. The board kept working to secure those large donations as well. They never took their foot off the fundraising gas pedal. They knew that for Ryan House to work long into the future, they needed to fundraise, fundraise, fundraise…

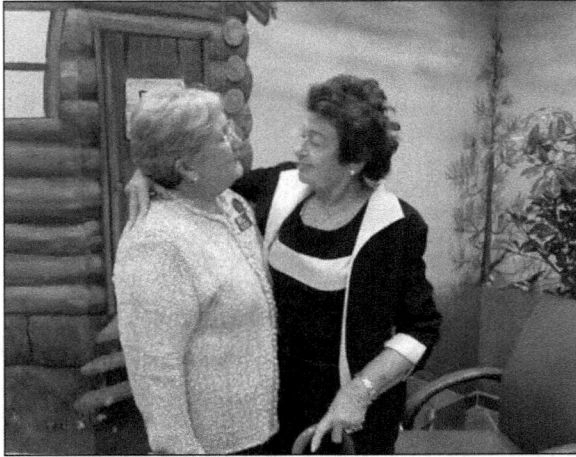

Judy Schubert and Gerda Weissmann Klein in the foyer of Ryan House

Author, Holocaust survivor, and 2011 Presidential Medal of Freedom recipient, Gerda Weissmann Klein, had been introduced to Ryan House by her close friend Judy Schubert by 2006. Nearing the opening, she offered to give the House a short story she had penned about her best friend. "Imagine a world in which your entire possession is one raspberry and you give it to your friend," the story begins. Gerda lived in that world. While in a Nazi concentration camp, her best friend Ilse discovered a single, bruised raspberry in a gutter on her way to the prison factory in which she worked. Knowing how much Gerda loved raspberries, Ilse scooped it up, stuck it in her pocket, and that night presented it to her best friend upon a single, dusty leaf she had plucked through the barbed wire.

When Judy heard the story, she immediately accepted the offer. She and other members of the board hired a local printer to produce the books. All of the proceeds from the sale of *One Raspberry* now support the endowment for Ryan House. But the book inspired so much more.

Suzanne Hanson wanted to give the house a bright, happy atmosphere where children would immediately feel at home. At George Mark Children's House she found each room had a different theme, with varied artwork and paint schemes. She liked the idea, but wanted to give it a distinctly Ryan

House feel. She invited a dozen local artists to a meeting where she explained the mission of the House and her vision for its interior design. The two went hand in hand. "We would like you to help us achieve this goal through your art. We're offering you the walls of the rooms as your canvases, with these children your audience. Here's the floor plan. Choose a room and show us what you would do."

After Suzanne spoke to the group, Gerda stepped forward. She told the story of the raspberry. If any artist needed added inspiration, this did it. The various artists came back a short time later with their portfolios. All the designs were different, with one exception: Every piece of art featured a single raspberry hidden within it.

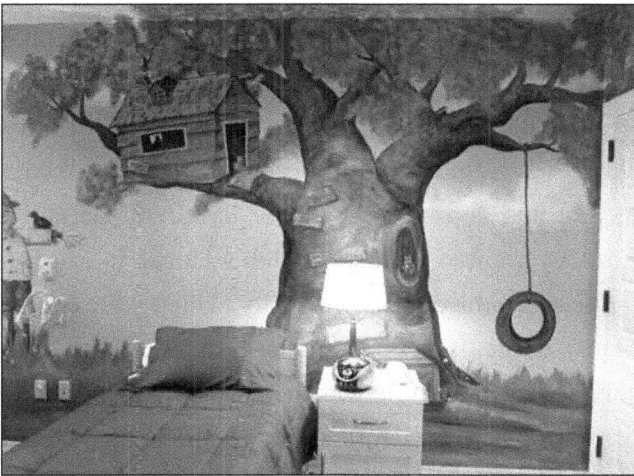

One of the eight children's rooms at Ryan House

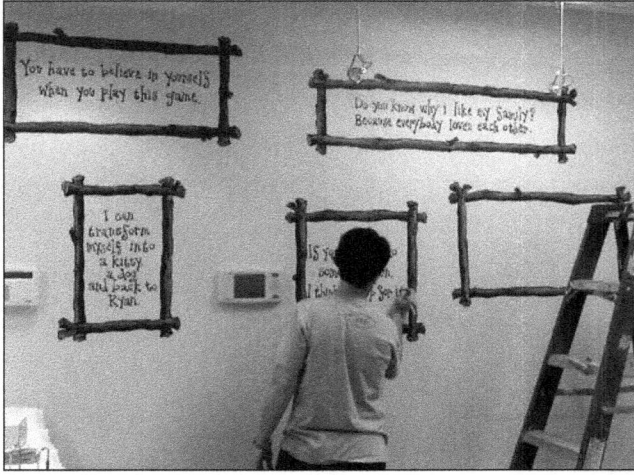

One of the many artists helping make Ryan House a home

While work progressed on construction of the house, a committee led by board members Connie Perez and Ginger Ward set out to formalize the care plan. Since Holly first sat down with Susan Levine and talked about starting a place for respite and end-of-life care for children, she and Jonathan had compared what they wanted to do with Helen House in England. They used words like respite and family and community, which were enough when Ryan House was mainly an idea. But now that the walls were going up, they needed something more concrete. Connie was the perfect person to ask for help.

Connie first came across Ryan House when she discovered the Run for Ryan House on the internet in 2007. Something about it grabbed her. She'd spent twenty-five years working in children's hospitals, most recently as the vice president of patient care at Phoenix Children's. She knew firsthand how sorely Ryan House was needed. As she read more about it, she told herself, "Wow, that's what I'd really like to do." She picked up her phone and called Nancy Martin. "How can I help?" she asked. At first she volunteered wherever needed. Before long, she was on the board of directors. After the house opened, she became its chair.

From the start, Connie focused on the operational aspects. When people talked about respite stays, Connie asked herself, "Okay, that sounds great, but what does it look like? What will the nurses do? What other types of staff do you need in the house? What roles do they need to fill?" While Hospice of the Valley had trained staff to do hospice care and even pediatric hospice care, this was different. Everyone involved wanted Ryan House to feel like going to grandma's house if grandma had lots of really cool stuff to do. "From the moment these kids come through the door, they need to feel like they've entered a place where they are totally loved and accepted. So how do we create that here?" she asked the board. She knew where to start to find the answer.

Earlier in her career, Connie managed the pediatric intensive care unit in a children's hospital in the Midwest. Late one night while working in the unit, she walked into the room of a ten-year-old boy dying from a brain tumor. He was awake and wanted to talk. "I don't know what to do," he said. "I know I am dying but my mom, she just doesn't want to accept it. I can't talk about it with her. Whenever I try she changes the subject or gets on to me saying I cannot give up. I haven't given up, but I know what's happening. I know I am dying. I just wish my mother would stop denying it."

"You're right," Connie said. "She doesn't want to believe it. But maybe together we can come up with a way for you to talk to her about it." The two of them came up with a plan which set the boy at ease. Two days later he died.

Fifteen years later, Connie remembered the conversation like it was yesterday. It reinforced to her the importance of a specialty known as child life in children's hospitals. Child life specialists focus on a child's emotional needs while connecting with the child on their level through honest conversations and especially through play. They set a child at ease and give them the freedom to open up in a very honest way about what they face. Like Connie's conversation with the boy in PICU, these are the conversations most haven't yet been able to have with their parents. Ryan House needed to be the safe place where these talks could take place. Holly and Jonathan fell in love with Helen House after their very open, honest conversation there with a doctor about dying and what that would one day look like with their son. Connie knew that finding the right child life specialists for Ryan House would help open the door for similar conversations, not only between adults but also between children and their parents.

The board agreed. Jenni Rogers, one of the child life specialists with whom Connie had worked at Phoenix Children's Hospital, had been active in the Ryan House Professional Services Committee for years and was passionate about supporting both children in their lifetimes as well as bereaved parents. "We need you over here," Connie had suggested in the past. When hiring began, Jenni enthusiastically applied and was hired with the title of Clinical Resource Coordinator – a staff role designed to enable her to continually support and promote child life.

Six months before the house was finished, long time Hospice of the Valley employee Pam Roman received a similar request. A registered nurse, she helped open HOV's second patient care home several years earlier. With Ryan House under construction, her boss and Ryan House board member Susan Levine came to her with a simple question, "How would you feel about leading the clinical team at Ryan House?"

Pam knew all about the House and she particularly liked the idea of working with the children and their families. As a hospice nurse, she'd worked with both adults and children. Over the years she'd found that she learned so many life lessons from children as they faced the end-of-life. "I think I would like that," she answered. "So what will that entail?"

"Well," Susan said, "it means you will need to build a team and then lead it for both the upstairs adult unit and downstairs for Ryan House. You have such a heart for these children. I think that makes you the perfect fit."

Pam loves challenges and the prospect of developing the care program appealed to her. "Count me in," she said.

Over the next several months she worked closely with Jenni Rogers and with Hospice of the Valley and Ryan House's Director of Operations, Sarah Bird, and Ryan House board members, Connie Perez and Ginger Ward, to develop the operational procedures for the House. They developed the criteria for those who would be eligible to use Ryan House, determined ways to get the word out to the families who needed their services and worked out the procedure for arranging for those families to actually stay at the House while making all the needed arrangements with their physicians. Through this entire process, she had to find a way to put these families at ease and reassure them that not only would their children be well cared for, they would also be loved.

Pam also had to assemble her care team, including nurses, certified nurse assistants, child life specialists, and social workers. Not just any team members would do. Working with hospice patients takes a very unique skill set, and working with pediatric hospice patients even more so. She set out to find staff with a passion for pediatrics and a deep empathy for families with children with life limiting conditions. Pam knew from experience how emotionally taxing Ryan House was going to be on its staff. One day her nurses would get to bake cookies with a child on a respite stay, and then at some point in the future, the nurse would find themselves caring for this child as they came to the end of the battle with their condition. Not everyone is cut out for such work. Pam was determined to find a child centered team that was.

They had time to bring the staff together. Construction stretched on for thirteen months. Working out the final details in terms of the house, staffing, and all the other details that had to be finalized soon began to wear down the team that had worked so long to make the dream of Ryan House a reality. Fatigue set in. Nerves grew short. Personalities clashed during board meetings. In the midst of one fourteen hour day, Nancy made up her mind that once the house was up and running, she would retire once and for all. Several board members rotated off, or made plans to step down. Yet, through it all, no one gave up. They kept pressing. Opening day was within sight.

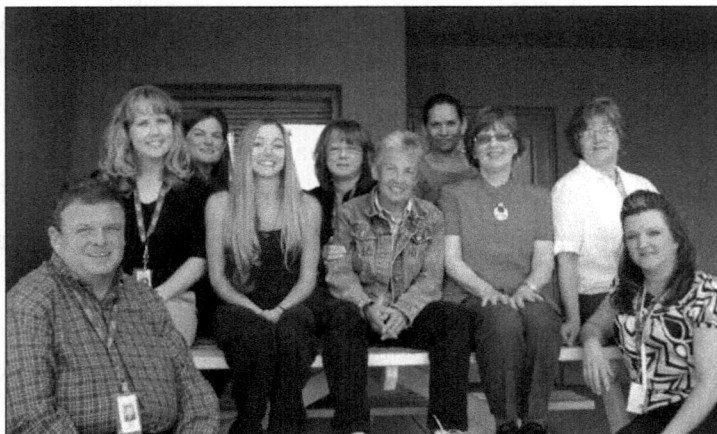

Ryan House's original world-class Care Team!

From left to right: Charley Coppinger, Jenni Rogers, Josie White, Amanda Thomas, Pam Roman, Joann "Jo" Ramundo, Maria Montufar, Roni Englett , Kasia Wojnarowska, and Helene Armstrong

In the Blink of an Eye

The opening of the baseball season and spring break came in the same week in 2007. Jonathan took Ethan and Ryan to a Diamondbacks game for a father / son night out. For a night, Jonathan forgot all about Ryan House and work and everything else that pulled him away from his sons even while he was with them. The three watched the game, ate hotdogs, and generally had the kind of time fathers and sons have been having at baseball games for generations.

However, Ryan had a little trouble enjoying the game because of an annoying cough that had been building for a few days. Kids and colds are nothing new, especially once they start school. However, Jonathan and Holly had to be extra careful with Ryan when he came down with anything. Ryan's SMA weakened his respiratory muscles, making it difficult for him to keep his lungs clear. As they learned when he was very young in England, a simple cold can quickly develop into pneumonia. Jonathan and Holly were diligent to keep that from happening again. They increased his chest physio treatments and treated his symptoms with medication. Aside from an annoyance, especially during his spring break, they were confident this cough would pass.

Two days later, Holly loaded up Ryan and Ethan in their van and headed off to Tucson ninety miles away. She wanted the boys to have a few days with her parents before they started back to school. Driving down Interstate 10 about forty five miles outside of Tucson, Ryan's temperature suddenly spiked. His breathing became very labored. Holly slammed her foot on the gas and flew down the highway. When she pulled into her parents' driveway, Budd walked out to meet them. "We've got to get Ryan to the hospital right away!" she yelled. She took Ethan inside for Judi to watch and made a quick call to Ryan's neurologist and asked which hospital they should go to and which doctors she should request. Budd jumped behind the wheel of her van and sped Holly and Ryan to University

Medical Center. The emergency room triage doctors rushed Ryan back and started IV antibiotics. He responded quickly, just as he always seemed to do. The hospital released him after a couple of hours. That night, Holly and the boys stayed with her parents as planned. However, the unplanned trip to the ER made her nervous. She cut their stay short and headed home the next morning.

Monday rolled around. Ryan still wasn't well enough to go back to school. Instead, his days were filled with breathing treatments every four hours all through the day and the night. A day or two later, Ryan awoke with another high fever. He could hardly breathe. Holly called Phoenix Pediatrics, his primary doctor's office, and told the nurse who answered the phone what was going on. A doctor immediately took the call. He walked Holly through how to test Ryan's capillary refill time. "I don't like the sound of this. Go ahead and bring him in right away," he told her.

Once she arrived at the Phoenix Pediatrics' office, the doctor who saw Ryan was visibly concerned. "We need to get him to the emergency room right away. You can either drive him or we can call an ambulance."

"Call the ambulance," Holly shot back. She quickly phoned a friend to go over to her house for Ethan who would soon return home from school. When the ambulance arrived, she climbed into the back with Ryan and headed off to Phoenix Children's Hospital. Dr. Tressia Shaw recommended he be taken to the Pediatric Intensive Care Unit (PICU) and be placed on bilevel positive airway treatment (BiPAP) to help his breathing. They started him on more IV antibiotics to treat the infection. This time there would be no quick release home. Jonathan joined Holly at the hospital. When he walked into his room he could not believe all the wires and tubes connected to his son. He flashed back to their day at the baseball game. It felt like a lifetime had passed instead of a few days.

The next morning, a respiratory therapist came into Ryan's room to give him his routine chest physio and breathing treatments. Jonathan had just stepped out to grab some coffee for the two of them. "How are you doing this morning, Ryan?" the therapist asked.

"He seems to be feeling better," Holly answered.

"Mom, I can talk for myself," Ryan chimed in.

"Sorry," Holly said.

"Moms are like that, aren't they," the therapist said as she sat Ryan up, started his chest vest and fitted his nebulizer mask. "Always doing all the talking for you." She started the machine.

"We can't help it. It's what we do. We're moms after all," Holly said with a laugh. Then she looked down at Ryan. His lips were moving, but no sound was coming out of his mouth. Suddenly, his eyes rolled back in his head and he stopped breathing completely. "HE'S GOT A PLUG! HE'S GOT A PLUG!" she yelled at the therapist, then ran into the next room to grab the nurse. Michael, the nurse working that day, ran in and went to work. He laid Ryan back and tried to clear his airway. Holly stayed by the door. She had to turn away. "Is this it?!" she couldn't help but think.

Time dragged by. Finally she saw Ryan's chest moving normally. Michael stepped back. "I think we got it. We've just got to make sure we clear all his airways before we start his breathing treatments."

About that time Jonathan sauntered into the room, a smile on his face and two cups of coffee in his hands. "Here you...go? What just happened?" he asked when he saw Holly's face drained of color. Holly could hardly tell him. The very thought that Ryan's condition could deteriorate so quickly left her shaken. Since his bout with pneumonia in England when he was very small, Ryan's health had been relatively good all things considered. The calm had lulled both of them into a sense of security. Yes, Ryan had SMA, but he was handling it. Every day he grew stronger and every day they learned ways to help him lead a full life in spite of his condition. The last ten minutes swept that sense of calm away. Reality had come back in a very big way.

Reality did not let up. While Ryan responded to the antibiotics, regular chest physio and newly added BiPAP, the incident with the mucus plug caused the doctors concern. On top of this, he was having trouble eating. While SMA can make it difficult to swallow, the real problem was Ryan's lack of an appetite. After a few bites he felt full. As a result, he wasn't getting nearly enough calories for a four year old boy.

A day or so after he was admitted, the PICU doctors pulled Holly and Jonathan aside. "We think it is time you seriously consider a trach for your son's breathing as well as inserting a G-tube. His breathing...well, you have seen that for yourself firsthand. And he's not getting the nutrition he needs orally. Both of these procedures will rectify the situation. As you well know, both are common for children with your son's condition."

"But he was fine a week ago," Jonathan protested. "I took him to a Diamondbacks game. He ate a hotdog. He didn't have any trouble swallowing that."

"We understand," one of the physicians replied. "But things can change quickly as you've witnessed these past couple of days. You don't have to make a decision today but you will need to make one soon."

After the doctors left, Jonathan and Holly stared at one another in disbelief. "Do we really have to have this conversation now?" Jonathan said. "I mean, if we cut his throat for the trach and insert the G-tube into his stomach, there's no going back. It's a slippery slope. What will come next? And what kind of quality of life will he have?"

Holly let out a long sigh. "How will he fit in with the other kids at school if we do this? He already stands out enough just with his chair and all the extra help he gets. But if we do this..." Her voice trailed off.

Neither one would say it but both thought back to their original conversations about letting nature take its course. How did trachs and G-tubes fit into that? They didn't want to even think about it.

This was not the last time one of the physicians talked to them about these two issues. Nor was it the last conversation Jonathan and Holly had about them. Both felt torn up inside, battered. The need to make a decision intensified five days into Ryan's hospital stay. He'd been transferred out of PICU and onto the respiratory floor. After much persuading, Jonathan finally convinced Holly to go home and get a decent night's sleep. She left around 5:30 in the evening. A short time later, Dr. Shaw checked on Ryan. As Jonathan placed Ryan's BiPAP mask on his face and started to tighten the straps, he joked, "It seems like we're finally out of the woods, Dr. Shaw." All of a sudden, Ryan's eyes rolled back in his head and his lips turned bright blue. Before Jonathan knew what was happening, Dr. Shaw hit the Code button on the wall, whipped off Ryan's BiPAP, leaped onto the bed and started CPR. To Jonathan, it seemed like half the hospital poured into the room. Before long, Ryan started breathing again and, yet again, all seemed clear. They transferred him back to the PICU. The next day, Jonathan and Holly enrolled in a CPR class offered at the hospital.

This second close call intensified the pressure on the Cottors to allow the doctors to insert the trach and G-tube. The afternoon after the incident, the two of them sat in Ryan's room, discussing what to do while Ryan slept. Michael, the nurse who saved Ryan's life a few days before, came in. Through his career, he spent a great deal of time caring for children in intensive care, especially pediatric palliative care. "I don't mean to intrude on your conversation," he said, "but I've heard what the doctors have suggested to you and I can see how torn up you are over this whole decision."

"That's an understatement," Jonathan replied.

"Listen, I've had opportunities to work with doctors involved with pediatric palliative care all over the country. I know you just want to do what is best for your son and I also think that you don't want to do anything invasive that will take away from his quality of life. I've always believed that, in a situation like this, the best thing you can possibly do is not to make a reactive decision. The doctors here, they just see what's happening right now and they're trying to fix it. That's what doctors are trained to do, and they're pretty good at it. But they don't know your journey. You do. You've lived it. You know it's okay if you just slow down and take this one step at a time. Instead of jumping right in with a trach, they can intubate him to help him get the air he needs. That may be all it takes right now. If it's not, then you can decide on a trach. But intubating him isn't a permanent step. The same with a G-tube. We can insert a nasal feeding tube for now. It's temporary and that may be all he needs. If it isn't, then you can make the call on a G-tube. The thing is, you don't have to take such big, permanent steps now. There are other options."

"That feels like such a relief, Michael," Holly said. "Thank you." Later that day Terri, a friend whose daughter, Destiny, also had SMA, dropped by the hospital. Holly filled her in on all that had happened, including their conversations with the PICU doctors about the trach and G-tube. "I've had that same conversation," Terri told them. "They wanted to do that to Destiny, but I just couldn't bring myself to do it, at least not so quick. So I said no."

"And she's fine now, right?"

"Yep," Terri said.

"Thanks. I know now what we're going to do."

After eighteen days, Ryan came home from the hospital without a trach and with only a temporary NG feeding tube. He turned five that week. Perhaps his greatest gift of all was that his family was able to remove the feeding tube the day before his party. After nearly losing him twice, both Jonathan and Holly treasured his birthday celebration. If they had ever been tempted to take these days for granted, they did not any longer. Once again, they were reminded that his condition could change in a moment. Every day with him was a gift.

Neither knew how many more gifts they would receive.

Section Three: A House Called Ryan

Chapter Eleven

Grand Opening

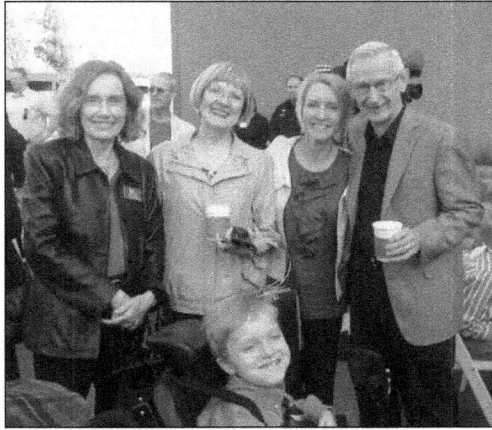

Diane Eckstein, Sharon, Holly, Bob, and Ryan
Cottor at the Ryan House opening

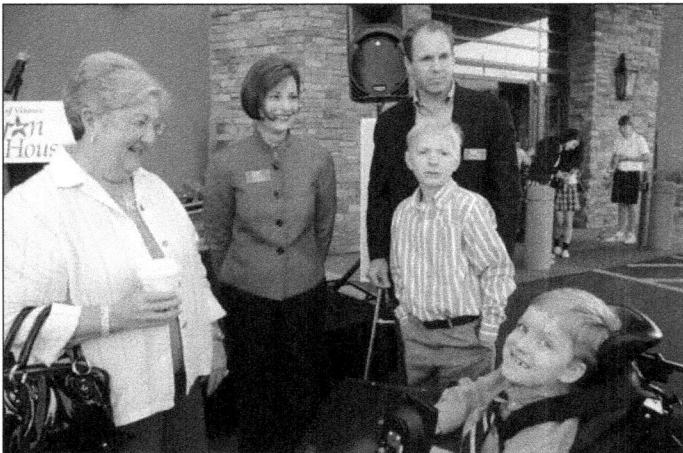

Judy Schubert, Judy Shannon, Jonathan, Ethan, and
Ryan Cottor at the Ryan House opening

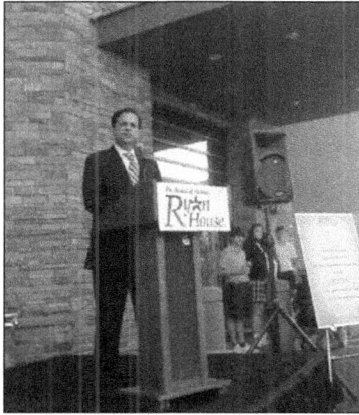

City of Phoenix Mayor, Phil Gordon

ON WEDNESDAY MORNING, MARCH 24, 2010, seven years after the Cottors moved to Phoenix from London, cameras flashed as Ryan Cottor took hold of one end of the rope that served as the Grand Opening ribbon across the Ryan House entrance. His brother, Ethan, grabbed the other end. Ryan pulled on the joystick he uses to steer his wheelchair. He inched backward, untying the knot and officially opening Ryan House. A reporter asked Ryan what he thought about getting to officially open the house named after him. "I thought it was only going to be an idea. I didn't think it would really happen," he replied.

Holly and Jonathan stood to the side and fought back tears. They never doubted the house would open, although they always feared Ryan would not live long enough to see it. That fear never really left them, even as the grand opening drew near. A few days earlier, Ryan had developed a respiratory infection. He appeared to be responding well to the latest round of antibiotics, but his many trips to the hospital had taught them to take nothing for granted.

"Are you going to stay in your house now that it's open?" a reporter asked Ryan.

"This isn't my house. It is as much my friend Madi's house or any kid who stays here's house."

"But are you going to stay here?" the reporter asked again.

"I think so," Ryan replied with a shrug of his shoulders.

After fulfilling his official duties, Ryan cruised back over to his mom. "I love Ryan House but I wish you'd called it something else. Everyone thinks I'm special because my name's on the sign and I'm not," he said.

"Oh, Ryan, you are special! You have done such a good job of being an ambassador for Ryan House. I know it hasn't been easy for you and I am SO proud of you. So many people are proud of you!"

"When we stay here, can I not be that Ryan? Can I just be the real Ryan and play and have fun?"

"Absolutely," Holly replied. She gave him a big hug.

"Mom," Ryan complained.

The rope untying ceremony was just one of many events leading up to actually opening the doors for families. A rope was chosen instead of the traditional ribbon cutting to go along with the house's interior decorating theme. After much back and forth with the board, Suzanne Hanson settled on a camp theme for every room to give children the feeling of "going off to camp" when they stayed there. The kitchen became the "S'more Café," while the hydrotherapy room, ie., the pool, became "The Swimming Hole." "Lake Squeaky Clean" was the bathing room while the music room was simply, "Do Re Mi." The cowboy camp theme included "Cowboy Ryan's" favorite quotes painted above the reception desk.

The official rope ceremony opened the doors, but the first guests would not arrive for a few days. First, the founders wanted to show the house off to all those who had a part in building it. Over the course of five days, Judy, Nancy and the board hosted different groups from the community that had given both time and money toward construction. Every day featured a special event tailored for the different groups. A celebratory mood marked every tour of the home, along with every speech thanking each group for their support. The CEO of one of Phoenix's largest banks, which had given $100,000 to the House, walked through the halls with Judy Schubert, tears of joy rolling down his face. "Oh my God," he said, "I never thought it would be anything like this. I am so happy you got us involved."

During the dedication ceremony, Nancy Martin, Judy Schubert and Judy

Shannon made speeches along with Phoenix Mayor Phil Gordon. "This is so beautiful, beyond anything we could have imagined," each one said. They talked about the location, thanking St. Joseph's, and they talked about the artwork in each room and the spacious, inviting entrances. As someone made another speech about how amazing all the special rooms were, Connie Perez leaned over to the Director of Inpatient Services, Sarah Bird, and whispered, "You watch. Next year at this time nobody is going to be talking about the House. All anyone will talk about are the kids and the families and what happens here."

She was right.

Ryan House officially opened for children on Monday, March 29, 2010. Edward and Diana Frieberg started the day rushing around their house, gathering the last of the items they needed for their son, Solomon, and daughter, Jessica's, overnight stay. Diana had come across an online ad for the House a few weeks earlier and called immediately. Pam Roman came to their home with brochures and explained the house's mission. To Edward and Diana, Ryan House sounded like an answer to a prayer. Ten years earlier they first became foster parents to a child with special medical needs. They later adopted the child. Through the years they fostered, then adopted nine other children, all with varying degrees of need. Jessie and Solly were the only two with diagnoses serious enough to qualify to stay at Ryan House.

For nearly a year, Edward and Diana had talked about taking their children to Disneyland, but they knew the trip would be more stressful than fun for Solly and Jessie. Ryan House presented the perfect solution. Diana planned on spending the first night there with them, then she and Edward and the rest of the kids would leave for Southern California.

After loading what appeared to be half of their house into their car, Edward walked back in the house and asked, "Do you think we have everything?"

"I've packed their clothes and diapers and formula and feeding supplies along with all their medications in their suitcase," Diana said.

"The suction machines, gait trainers, standers, pulse oximeters and oxygen bottles are in the van."

"The oxygen company is supposed to deliver bottles directly to Ryan House," Diana reminded Edward.

"I know. But I still packed a couple of extra bottles just in case."

"That's a good idea." Diana looked around and let out a little sigh. "Okay. I think I have everything."

"Looks like more than everything to me," Edward said.

"It probably is but you can never be too careful. After all, they're going to be there for an entire week," Diana said. "I guess that's it. I'm on my way." As soon as she left, Edward went back to packing for their Disneyland vacation.

All the dignitaries and special visitors had left by the time Diana walked through Ryan House's front door on Monday morning. She and Jessie and Solly were officially the House's very first guests. (The Cottors joined them a few hours later.) The House exceeded her expectations. "Wow," she said as she walked in. "Wow, wow, wow."

A familiar face greeted her. "Diana, I'm so glad to see you again," Pam said. She crouched down to get on eye level with Jessica in her chair. "We have so much planned for your stay, Jessie. I'm so happy you and your brother are staying with us. Are you ready to have some fun?" Jessie lit up. Although unable to respond verbally, it was clear how she loved the personal attention.

"So, Diana, let's get the three of you settled into your rooms." Pam led the three of them down the left hand hallway. "Jessie this is your room," she said as they came to the first bedroom. "Solly, you're going to be right next door."

"Does it matter which of the two rooms I land in?" Diana asked.

"You aren't staying in either of the children's rooms. It wouldn't be much of a respite for you if you did. We have a very nice suite for you right down this hall." Pam pointed to the small hall that ran past the reception desk.

"I just thought this first night you would want me in there with them."

Pam smiled. "You are welcome to spend as much time with your children to help our staff get to know both of them. I think you will enjoy that. But make sure you take some time for yourself. We'll take good care of Jess and Solly."

As Pam and the staff settled Jessica and Solomon into their rooms, Diana pulled her suitcase down the short hall and opened the door to her room. "Oh my. I didn't know I was going to get to visit a resort tonight," she said. The room featured everything she hoped to find in a very nice hotel room: Flat screen television, artwork, an inviting queen sized bed covered with pillows and a private patio where she could sit and read. "Edward missed out by staying home. I may stay here and skip Disney. This beats a hotel room with eight kids."

She rejoined her children as Nurse Roni pushed Solly into the "Sensory Tent", which is not a tent at all but the first room down the right hand hall next to the S'more Café. Diana had never seen anything like it. Few outside of those who have stayed at Ryan House or places like it in England or George Mark Children's House ever have. The room itself was awash with lights, sounds, colors and different textures that stimulate a child's senses. A mat covered the center of the room. From above, a projector shone down images on the mat, images that responded whenever Solly reached out and tried to touch them. His eyesight is limited to mainly colors and indistinct shapes but that didn't stop him from reaching his hand into the ocean as it danced on the mat before him. Diana choked up. This was the closest her son had ever come to the beach, or probably ever could because of his physical limitations.

Next door, Robert, one of the volunteers, pressed a maraca into Jessica's hand. "Like this?" he said as he shook it while holding her hand. She rocked back and forth, moving her entire body as she made the maraca sing. The volunteer clapped. "That's the way. You're rocking it, Jessie."

Pam appeared in the music room doorway. "We have a surprise for you," she said.

An older man came in behind her carrying a banjo. "Well hello little lady," he said. "Looks like you like music. Do you mind if I play a little for you?"

Diana spoke up. "She would love it, but hold on just one minute. Let me go get my son."

She ran next door, then returned with Solomon. For the next fifteen minutes, Diana, Jessica and Solomon sat transfixed by the music. After their private concert, Diana thanked the banjo player over and over. "It truly is my privilege to come here and play for your kids," he replied. "I'm glad this place is finally open so that I can come. I've been waiting to do this for a very long time."

The Cottors arrived shortly after the concert ended. Jonathan opened the door for Holly and the boys, then paused before walking through himself. "What's wrong?" Holly asked.

"I've walked through these doors so many times during construction and even last week for all the grand opening ceremonies but it never felt like this."

"It's surreal, isn't it? Ryan said it best this morning when he said it always just seemed like an idea we kept chasing that would never actually happen."

"I knew it would happen."

"I did, too. I just mean that it seemed so out there, almost like a dream. To finally walk through the doors as a family for a stay, well, it's just," Holly's voice cracked, "it's almost too much to believe."

"Are you two coming in or what?" Ethan said with an annoyed tone.

Jonathan laughed. "Yeah, we're right behind you!"

The staff led the Cottors to Ryan's room. Because of his respiratory infection, his room was on the opposite end of the house from Jessica and Solomon. Under normal circumstances, he would not have been able to stay at all until he was completely recovered. But this was not a normal circumstance. On top of that, the Cottors and Friebergs were the only families scheduled to stay during the opening week. Pam Roman decided they could make an exception just this one time.

"So where do you want to stay?" Pam asked Ethan.

"I get to pick?" Ethan replied. "I thought I had to stay with my mom and dad?"

"No. Not this week. Pick a room and it's yours. You get to break one in and be the very first guest to use it. See if you can spot the raspberry!"

He looked around. "I like this one," he said pointing to the room right next door to his brother. The mural included a campfire scene on one wall. "Yep, this is the one!"

Holly and Jonathan went to their suite. A fresh arrangement of daffodils sat on the nightstand, with an envelope propped up next to it with their names on the front. Inside they read, "Dear Holly and Jonathan, Thank you for all the light and sunshine you have brought to so many children and families. I hope your weekend has been memorable. Love, Jan." The note came from Jan Johnson who had coached the capital campaign committee that raised the money to make this room possible. "I wish Jan was here," Holly said, handing the card to Jonathan. "She was a HUGE part of that light. We wouldn't be here if it weren't for her. Or at least, not yet."

Ethan and Ryan immediately ventured into the living room equipped with a fifty inch flat screen television complete with both Wii and Xbox game systems. Before they could boot up a game, they heard some sort of commotion coming from outside in the hall. "What the?" Ethan said. The two boys turned around just as Darth Vader and an Imperial storm trooper came walking in.

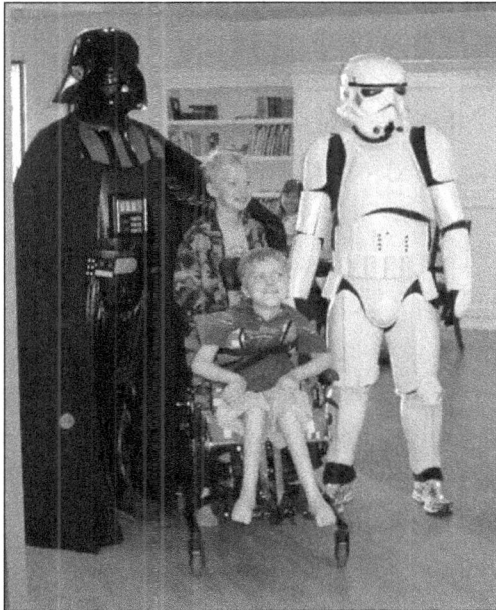

From left: Darth Vader, Ethan, Ryan, and a
Storm Trooper at Ryan House

"Where is Skywalker?" Vader demanded. "I know you two know where he is hiding. Give him up to me."

"We don't know where he is," Ryan said.

"You rebel scum. Tell me where he is!"

"He was here, but he left," Ryan said. "He left the planet. I think he was going back to Tatooine."

"For your sake, I hope he is," Vader said with a menacing tone. He spun on his heels and headed out the door, the storm trooper close behind him.

"Tatooine?" Ethan said in a mocking tone.

"Hey, I had to say something to keep Luke safe," Ryan replied.

Holly and Jonathan rejoined their sons after Vader left. "So what do you boys want to do first?" Jonathan asked. Both he and Holly felt like they needed to dive right in and experience everything the house had to offer.

"We kind of wanted to chill for a while, if that's okay," Ethan said. "Besides, we were just about to play a video game."

"You have those at home," Jonathan replied. "Come on. There's a lot to do and see here. Let's check out the sensory room."

Ethan let out an annoyed sigh.

"You want to shoot video?" Holly asked Ethan. "One of the board members gave Ryan House a flip video camera the other day so you can make a movie of your stay. This would be a great time to try it out."

Ethan dropped the video controller. "Sure. Okay. Whatever."

"I want to swim," Ryan said. Ryan always enjoys swimming because the water is the one place his arms and legs work the way they are supposed to.

"Let's get our suits on," Jonathan said. Holly started to go with Ryan to help him change clothes but Rachel, one of the nurses, stepped into the room. "I can help Ryan get ready. Ready buddy? I felt the water earlier and it is just right, Ryan. You will love it!"

"Let's go!" Ryan said.

After swimming, the four spent the rest of the evening in the kitchen, cooking together. "Make sure you video this," Jonathan told Ethan.

"I don't think future generations are going to get all stoked about you boiling water, dad," Ethan said.

"You know what I mean," Jonathan said.

Ethan shot a few moments of video, then said to Ryan, "Come on, let's go outside and mess around." The two shot toward the door.

"Boys," Jonathan said.

"Let them go have fun," Holly said. "We can cook together at home, too. It's not that big of a deal."

"I know but it kind of is. We have never cooked HERE. We're the first people to ever use this kitchen." He looked around. "I wish other families were in here like at Helen House. I think it is very important that we recreate that atmosphere here."

"Give it time," Holly said.

Later that evening, the two of them settled into their suite. "So what do you think?" Jonathan asked.

"You mean about the house? It's great."

"Yeah it is. But I was a little concerned when we first got here. Settling in wasn't nearly as smooth as it was at Helen House."

"But they've been at it for over twenty five years," Holly said. "This is Ryan House's first day."

"I guess. I also miss the interaction with other families that we had over there. We barely had a chance to even say hi to Diana."

"That's because we were trying to do everything in the first day. Relax. This isn't Helen House. It's Ryan House. It's going to take on its own personality. I'm sure all the children's hospices in England each have their own distinct feel."

"You're right." He paused for a very long time. Finally he said, "Can you believe we are actually staying here? We're really here. Wow. Six years of work and we're finally here with our boys." The two laid in the silence, soaking in the moment.

Diana Frieberg awoke the next morning more than a little disoriented. It was her first full night's sleep in nearly ten years. No monitor alarm bells went off. No child cried for her in the night. She didn't have to turn anyone over and check on their breathing. She wasn't sure what to do with herself.

She flipped on the television and watched a little of a morning news program. Bored with it quickly, she went out into the hall. Staff members surrounded both of her children, playing with them, fussing over them, treating them like they were their own. "They're getting pampered like they are at a five star resort," she said to no one in particular. "That's what this place is. It's a resort for special needs children." She headed toward the kitchen to make herself a cup of coffee. Walking past the reception desk, she stopped to talk to Pam. "You know, when word gets out about this place, you're going to have your hands full. There are a lot of families out there who are going to go nuts over Ryan House."

"That's what we're hoping for," Pam said.

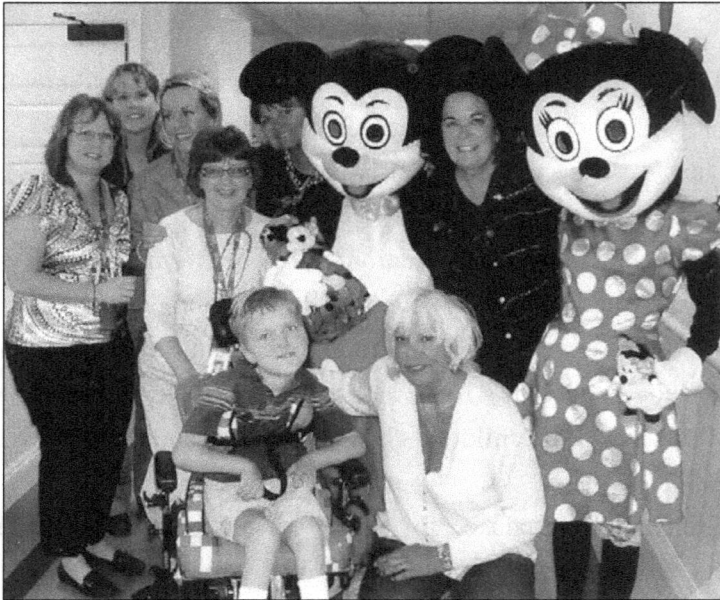

Mickey and Minnie come to visit Ryan and staff at Ryan House

Diana spent some time with her children before leaving to join the rest of her family for their Disneyland adventure. After she left, Pam and the Ryan House staff took her children's experience up to a whole different level. Pam knew the rest of the family was headed to the Magic Kingdom but she didn't want Jessie and Solly to miss out completely. She arranged for a special visit for the two of them from two of their favorite Disney characters, Mickey and Minnie Mouse. The children lit up when their favorite celebrities walked in the door just for them.

But they weren't their only visitors. Like every little girl, Jessica loved princesses, especially Disney princesses. After Mickey and Minnie left, Snow White came into her room. Jessica is confined to a wheel chair and is non-verbal, but she let everyone know how excited she was to meet Snow White. Later, a volunteer named Alice helped dress Jessica in a princess costume. Pam put on a CD of Disney princess songs. As the music played, this non-verbal child began to sing while moving her shoulders around, dancing in her wheelchair.

When Diana and Edward saw the photographs in the children's memory books after they returned, Diana shook her head and smiled. "Yep, when word gets out these rooms will always be full." Pam gave her the Disney CD. Jessica still sings and dances every time they play it for her.

Morgan

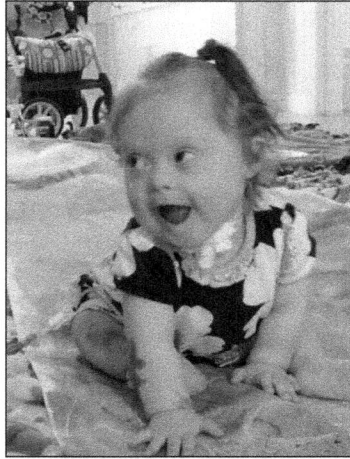

Morgan

Pam Roman walked past the reception area as the phone rang. "Hey, Pam, it's for you. It's Morgan's dad."

"Great," Pam said. "It's about time he calls to make a reservation for her. We haven't seen her in a while. I really miss that girl. We need to get her in while we still can."

Over the previous two years, Morgan had become not only one of Pam's favorites but the favorite of most of the staff and volunteers. Her family utilized their full allotment of twenty eight days at the house each year, which helped all the staff feel very close to her. Only three years of age, Morgan had already overcome a great deal of adversity. Born with Downs Syndrome and a complete Atrioventricular Canal defect, her parents feared she would not survive her first year. The surgery to correct her heart condition, which consisted of a hole in the wall between the two sides in the middle of her heart, weakened her already weak lungs to the point that she needed a ventilator to stay alive. However, not long after her first birthday she grew strong enough for another round of surgery that not only completed the repairs to her heart but also allowed her to come off the ventilator. As time went by, she improved to a point where Pam had already started talking to her parents about the very real possibility that Morgan might no longer meet the criteria for Ryan House stays.[6] That is why she was excited to hear from Morgan's dad. Pam wanted to get Morgan in as many times as she could while she still qualified.

"Hi, Phillip, it's great to hear from you," Pam said.

"Yeah. Hi Pam." Pam could tell from the tone of his voice that something was wrong. "I just called...Uh. Yeah." There was silence on the phone for a few moments followed by a long sigh. "Uh, Morgan's in the PICU over at Phoenix Children's and she's...uh..." Another sigh. "She's not doing so good."

"Oh, Phillip, I'm so sorry."

"Yeah, thanks, uh, Jess and I were wondering if some of you could maybe come over to the hospital. We could, uh, you know, really use some help right now."

"Absolutely. Yes. We'll be right there."

"I really appreciate it. You know, Morgan loves Ryan House. And if she," another long pause, "if it looks like she isn't going to make it, we want to bring her there. I don't want her to die in a hospital. I want her in a place she loves and that makes her happy."

Pam choked back tears. How is this possible? She was doing so well. "We will do whatever you need us to do. We can talk more when I get to the hospital. I will be there very soon."

Pam hung up the phone and bent over as if she'd been hit in the stomach. Karina, the staff member who had originally answered the phone, looked at her with shock. "Oh no. What happened?"

"Morgan is sick and they aren't sure if she's going to make it."

"No, no, oh my God, no."

Pam found Jenni Rogers and told her what had happened. "I'll go

with you," Jenni said. Pam notified Veronica, one of the social workers who worked both with Ryan House and the pediatric units of the
area hospitals, and asked her to meet them at Phoenix Children's
Hospital. On her way to her car, Pam also called Rachel Colwell,
one of the nurses who had worked at Ryan House since its opening.
Rachel had built a strong relationship with Morgan and her parents.
She was off on this particular day. "Rachel, it's Pam. I just got a call
from Morgan's dad. She's in the PICU at Phoenix Children's and it
sounds really bad. I knew you would want to know. I'll call with an
update after I assess the situation at the hospital."

Pam, Jenni and Veronica arrived at the hospital not long after Phillip
called. They found Morgan's room. Her two older sisters fidgeted at
the door while their grandparents tried to keep them in the hallway.
"Hey girls," Veronica said, "Why don't you come with me for a little
while?" The girls looked up at their grandparents. Their grandfather nodded his assent. Veronica took them down to the waiting
area where she pulled out some puzzles from a bag and kept them
occupied.

Entering Morgan's room, Pam immediately recognized the severity
of the situation. The doctors had placed Morgan on an oscillating
ventilator (OVP), which meant she was on full life support. The girl
in the bed hardly looked like the same little girl who squealed and
giggled through her weekends at Ryan House.

"The doctors aren't very hopeful," Jessica, Morgan's mother, said.
"When we first brought her in they said she had pneumonia but then
all her organs just started shutting down. They can't tell us why."

"Jessica, I am so sorry. Morgan is such a precious little girl," Pam
said. She and Jenni stayed with the family for most of the afternoon, watching Morgan and sharing Ryan House memories with
mom and dad.

"You know, her sisters loved staying there as much as Morgan did,"
Jessica said. "They always got very jealous when Morgan went
by herself and we didn't stay as a family. It didn't matter where we
were going for vacation. The girls wanted to all stay at Ryan House.
That's why they loved the parties you guys have there. Everyone
got to go then. But usually only Morgan got to spend the night.

We told the older two that it was Morgan's special place." Jessica smiled for the first time since Pam and Jenni arrived. "She really loves it there. And she really loves that playground. It is one of the only playgrounds she can really use."

"You don't know how much Ryan House means to us," Phillip said. "That's why, if the doctors say she definitely isn't going to make it, we're bringing her there. It's like home to her."

Shortly after Rachel arrived at work the next day, Pam came and found her. "Morgan's condition deteriorated last night. They want to move her here. Frankly, she probably won't survive being taken off the OVP and placed on a vent that will get her here. Her parents understand, which is why they called. They would like for us to be there when they remove the vent, just in case." Pam, Rachel and a child life specialist named Kristen went back to the hospital. Like the day before, Morgan's older sisters fidgeted with their grandparents. Kristen took them and their grandparents into another room. They played together, play that was designed to help the girls work through what they were feeling with their sister.

Pam and Rachel walked into Morgan's room. Jessica greeted them with long hugs. A team of doctors and nurses hovered over Morgan. "They're going to try to switch her over to a vent we can use to move her," Jessica said. "But they don't know..." She couldn't finish the sentence. She didn't need to. Pam and Rachel understood.

Jessica and Phillip stayed as close as they could to their daughter while the medical team worked. Rachel stood back just a little, giving everyone space and wondering if she should even be there. A voice in her head kept telling her to leave, that she had intruded on a very private moment. She stayed anyway.

The process of switching Morgan from the OVP only took a few minutes but to everyone in the room it felt like hours. The nurse in Rachel kept wanting to jump in and help but she stayed back. You're here for mom and dad. You're here for mom and dad, she told herself over and over. She could hardly take seeing Morgan like this.

Once the medical team switched Morgan off the OVP and onto a travel ventilator, they stepped back for a moment and watched the monitors. Everyone in the room held their breath, not sure what might happen next. The monitors blinked and clicked the way they are supposed to. "It looks like she's stable," the doctor said. With that, all of the hospital staff left the room.

Jessica and Phillip stood there, each holding Morgan's hands, looking intently at their daughter. Then Jessica looked over at Rachel. "What now? Does this mean we can move her?"

All of Rachel's apprehension about intruding on a private moment evaporated. She stepped up, put her arm around Jessica, and explained what was next. "It looks like she is stable enough on the vent to transport. So I'm going to go over to Ryan House right now and get everything ready for her so that she will be comfortable as soon as we get her settled in there."

"I'll stay with you until the paramedics arrive to move her," Pam said.

"Thank you," Phillip said. "That sounds good. If she has to die, she's going to die at Ryan House."

At Ryan House, Rachel enlisted Kasia to help get Morgan's room ready. She'd stayed there so many times in the past that they knew how she liked her room. Kasia placed a bright, pink and purple blanket on the bed, and surrounded it with brightly colored pillows. She arranged some of Morgan's favorite toys over to one side, even though she knew there was no need for them. More than anything, she wanted the room to look and feel like it did the last time Morgan stayed for respite.

While Kasia prepared the room, Rachel gathered all the medications she needed to remove Morgan from the ventilator. In this situation, the single most important thing to mom and dad was that their little girl was comfortable and pain free. Dr. Tressia Shaw, one of the pediatricians who worked closely with Ryan House, arrived before the family. She and Rachel discussed the procedure but this was more of a formality. The two had worked with families under the same circumstances several times. However, Rachel found preparing the room for Morgan to be very difficult emotionally. She'd been trying to prepare herself emotionally for Morgan leaving Ryan House because she was too healthy to stay there any longer. No one, absolutely no one, ever thought this could happen.

The ambulance arrived a half hour after Rachel. Paramedics moved Morgan down the hallway to one of the rooms at the end of the hall across from the sanctuary room. These two rooms are primarily used for end-of-life care, not respite. Mom and dad lifted her from the gurney and sat down on the bed, holding her. Other family members gathered in the room as well, including grandparents, siblings and extended family. Rachel and Dr. Shaw sat down on the day bed next to the bed where Jessica and Phillip held Morgan.

Finally, Jessica looked over at Rachel and whispered, "Okay."

Rachel stepped over and removed the tube connecting Morgan to the ventilator. She then switched off the machine as well, making the room very quiet. Unlike the hospital, Rachel did not feel uneasy about being in the room in this moment. She knew the family wanted and needed her there. As Jessica and Phillip held their daughter, stroking her face and telling her how much they loved her, Morgan died. A look of complete peace came over her face. Her fight was over. Jessica wrapped her in her favorite blanket and held her tight.

Rachel excused herself. Quickly, she went to the restroom next to the reception desk and closed the door behind her. All the emotions she'd kept bottled up came pouring out. She then washed her face and went back to the family.

After the family had spent as much time as they needed with Morgan, a funeral director stepped into the room. "Whenever you are ready. We have the cot here we can place her on."

"Do you think it would be okay if I carry her out myself?" Jessica asked.

The funeral director looked over at Rachel as if to say, "Your call."

"Yes. Absolutely," Rachel replied.

Jessica stood, her daughter wrapped tight in her arms and carried her out through the back door to the waiting van. After she placed Morgan safely inside, Jessica stepped back. Her aunt came and put her arm around her shoulders. "When you insisted on bringing her here I could not understand why. Now I do," the aunt said.

"It's her place," Jessica said softly. "It always will be."

Chapter Twelve

Growing Pains

THE FIRST FAMILY TO COME to Ryan House for end-of-life care arrived when the house had been open for less than a week. A mom had dropped her little girl off at day care that morning. A few hours later she and her husband found themselves staring into the faces of doctors telling them there was nothing more that could be done for their child. The girl who started the day dancing into day care without a care in the world had choked on a cracker, but no one noticed until it was too late. Paramedics revived her long enough to get her to the hospital where she was placed on a ventilator. Tests revealed her brain had gone far too long without oxygen for her to survive. Her parents agreed to remove her from the ventilator. To their surprise, the girl kept breathing on her own. The hospital called Ryan House. "Can you accommodate this family and all their extended family?" A short time later, all the Ryan House rooms and family suites filled up with grandparents and aunts and uncles and cousins. People slept on the sofa in the great room and on the couches and chairs in the sanctuary. Charley, the Ryan House chaplain that everyone referred to as Charley Chaplain, arrived a short time later. He rarely left the family's side until the girl died a few days later.

For Nancy Martin, the first end-of-life care family was a sober reminder of the house's dual purpose. All the joy she felt during the Grand Opening celebrations and the excitement of watching the Cottors and Friebergs enjoy the house for respite gave way to grief watching this family suffer. *It's why we built it,* she told herself. *If we weren't here, where would they go? Where else could so many people spend so much time saying goodbye without worrying about disturbing anyone else?*

In the weeks that followed other families came and went, both for respite and end-of-life care. The house began to function exactly like the founders had envisioned. Seeing the operation working reassured Nancy the decision she'd made before the doors ever opened, was the right one. She formally submitted her resignation to the board of directors. "I'll stick around until you find a replacement," she told Judy Schubert.

A few weeks later board chair Judy Shannon came to her with a gift. "I'm giving you your summer, Nancy. I know these past three years have taken their toll on you and we very much appreciate all you've done. We couldn't have built this without you. I know you have a new grand baby on the way and you have a lot to do to get ready for its arrival. So you don't have to stick around until your replacement arrives in the fall. You can take off now if you like."

Nancy packed up and left by the end of the week. She'd put off retirement for three years for Ryan House. She didn't want to put it off any longer.

Other changes soon followed. In the six years it took Ryan House to go from concept to open for business, the board of directors swelled from the original eight to sixteen. However, even with what everyone considered to be an amazing collection of talent, the strain of getting the house built as well as the fatigue from the years of non-stop fundraising left many members drained. Now that the House was open, the board began to transition. From the start, board policy stated board members could serve no more than two consecutive three year terms without taking at least a one year sabbatical. Many of the original board members including Judy Schubert and Jonathan had to rotate off the year Ryan House opened. Neither was thrilled with stepping down at what they considered to be a crucial time but they knew the policy was a good one. It kept the board fresh, bringing in new members, which also broadened the house's community support.

Not only did the membership of the board begin to change, so did its focus. Now that the House was up and running, they shifted from a capital campaign to creating a fundraising process capable of cultivating significant donations for the long term day-to-day operations. Originally, the board members came together with the passion to get the House built and functioning. Early meetings had taken place in Diane Eckstein's living room, complete with homemade cookies. It was a very organic, grassroots movement, composed of members experienced in getting things done. Many had very strong personalities that would not take no for an answer, the very people a board must have to launch such a project from nothing.

However, as the board shifted its focus from building the house to sustaining it long term, the leadership team realized that any new members needed a different skill set. While the original board had raised seven million dollars in six years, every current and future board of directors had to raise more than $1.8 million *every year* to keep the House up and running.

For the first year of operations, the board decided to limit the House to only fifty percent of its capabilities. Since this was such a new concept for families to understand and become comfortable with, the Care Team knew it would take time to build a level of trust with qualifying families for them to fully utilize the house. Second, starting off slow gave the board time to gain momentum on the operational fundraising programs. This also gave the Care Team time to more fully develop its processes and culture as the program was new to everyone.

The slow start didn't last long. Word quickly got out to families and the demand started fast. The house reached one hundred percent usage sooner than anyone anticipated, along with the need to raise $2.5 million annually. Because the House offered its services at no charge to families, all of this money had to be raised through the generosity of the community.

The mindset of the board and the community now needed to change. Rallying to build the House had a clear objective and timetable. Once the House was finished, once the ribbon was cut (or, in this case, the rope untied) and the last speech was made, there was, as always occurs, a natural sigh followed by "now what?" The challenge had always been to not only build the House, but to create an ongoing sustainable care model for the long-term. It was important for all to stay focused and maintain momentum.

The board faced the challenge of convincing the community that the work had only begun with the opening of Ryan House. They needed Phoenix not only to rally to build it, but also to give, to make it possible for the children and families to continue to use the House. The transition from raising money as part of a capital campaign to shifting to an ongoing approach wasn't always as smooth as everyone had hoped it would be. Some of the longtime board members stepping down raised red flags within the community, requiring those who took their place to spend much of their time rebuilding relationships. Every nonprofit start up experiences similar growing pains but that knowledge didn't make the task of fundraising any easier for the new board members.

The House also experienced turnover in its executive staff. Within a year after Nancy's replacement was hired, the board found itself searching for a new Executive Director once again. They also had an instability with the Development Director position, a key position when it comes to fundraising. Again, Ryan House wasn't the first nonprofit to go through this sort of turnover early in its existence which is why the original board insisted on banking three years of operating capital before opening the doors. That cushion gave the board the time to get things right.

No matter what happened behind the scenes with the board and the executive staff, the House grew into a vital part of the community. More and more pediatricians recommended Ryan House to their patients. The special needs community also started talking about the House. Diana Frieberg wasn't the only mom who talked about how great Ryan House was for her kids. Every family that stayed there talked about it with their friends. Before long, Pam and the others in charge of the schedule faced a problem: More families wanted to use the House than they could accommodate at one time.

The more frequently a child stays and the family utilizes Ryan House, the stronger the connection becomes and the more support they feel. Following the example of children's hospices in the UK, Ryan House set a limit of twenty-eight days per year per family. That could be a weekend a month or perhaps up to a week at a time, whatever worked well for the family. With only eight children's bedrooms, families realized they had to share this resource to make it work. Even with the limit, the house's popularity kept growing.

As the use of the House grew, the staff soon discovered one area of the House remained strangely empty. Although every family is required to stay in one of the family suites the first time a child stays in the house, very few used the suites after their initial visit. Most families dropped their children off at Ryan House alone after that. The family rooms were being used during a child's end-of-life period, rarely for planned respite stays. While that speaks to the trust these families had with the Care Team, it also made it difficult to develop the sense of community Jonathan and Holly had experienced in England. More than anything, they wanted families in Phoenix to experience the same kind of connection at Ryan House. But, if no one ever stayed beyond their required time, how could they possibly create that sense of community?

The answer appeared without anyone really realizing they had found it. Ryan House opened in late March, 2010. When Halloween rolled around seven months later, someone had an idea: Let's have a party for all our kids and let them all dress up in costumes and have a great time. And if we're going to invite the kids, we should also invite their siblings. And if we're going to invite the kids and their brothers and sisters, mom and dad need to come as well. The Halloween party was such a hit that the staff decided to have a Holiday party in December. A few months later, they had a Spring party. Everyone seemed to enjoy the parties so much that someone on staff suggested having a movie night. The first movie night led to more reasons to hold parties and events for the families. Some did not include all families, such as the Mother's Day brunch they held for the single moms connected to the House.

In the midst of all the parties and celebrations, something dynamic happened. People started connecting with one another. The sense of family and community the founders hoped to build through families staying at the house began to grow through a completely different avenue. While this wasn't the way that anyone had originally envisioned, it didn't matter. Gatherings are part of what make Ryan House uniquely its own.

Pam and her Care Team also discovered that the level of care they needed to provide to their children exceeded their original expectations. When the English children's hospices, upon which Ryan House is modeled, started their work in the early 1980's, very few children needed high levels of technical care. It was rare to see a child living with a ventilator. However, with advances in treatment for chronic illnesses over the past few decades, more and more children survive longer with conditions that would have proved fatal in earlier generations. Hospice of the Valley also did not have much experience with acute care, even in its pediatric units. Children who used their services prior to HOV's partnership with Ryan House only came to HOV for end-of-life care, which required a lower staffing level than acute care.

As more and more families came to Ryan House, the staff discovered many of the children required far more personal care than they had anticipated. Not all of the nurses were comfortable doing this. Those who were used to providing hospice care were at times ill at ease working with a child with a trach on a ventilator. At the same time, some who were very skilled and comfortable providing a high level of care were not as comfortable with end-of-life care. It took some time for the team to become completely comfortable with both.

On top of this, because of the number of high need children coming for respite, Pam needed more staff on hand than she had originally anticipated. More and more children needed one-on-one care, which made Ryan House even more dependent on their team of volunteers to help meet this need. Thankfully, the partnership with Hospice of the Valley provided fantastic resources and processes to recruit, train, and oversee the wonderful volunteers. While the Care Team staff is always responsible for the care of the children while at Ryan House, volunteers are integral to help cook meals, play, and generally support the day-to-day running of the house.

From the start, the staff also found the families whose children have died at Ryan House continued to need their support long after that death. Obviously, as a children's *hospice* connected to one of the largest non-profit hospices in the nation, everyone knew going in that families who came for end-of-life care would need support afterward. Hospice of the Valley provides bereavement counselors for the families for the first two years after their child's death. But Ryan House took this a step further. Once a family becomes part of the Ryan House family, they're in the family as long as needed.

In addition, Ryan House built a memorial garden directly off of the sanctuary room for the families whose children die there. The idea came from the children's hospices in England. A grant paid for a local artist, who just so happened to have a child who regularly came to Ryan House for respite care, to create ceramic tiles for the garden wall. Each family chooses what they want the tile to be, with most choosing butterflies or dragonflies with the child's name etched upon them. However, no one ever anticipated the depth of connection families feel to those tiles. As more and more tiles dotted the garden walls, families began dropping by, many just sitting and staring at the butterfly on the wall. Almost all take photographs of the tiles, with some families taking family portraits in front of them.

As increasingly more families dropped by to spend time in the garden, Jenni Rogers made a suggestion. "Let's hold a memorial service and invite all the families whose child has died at Ryan House since we opened, to attend." At that time there were already forty tiles on the wall. To everyone's surprise, almost all the families showed up on Sunday afternoon for the service. As Jenni walked down the hall toward the sanctuary room and the garden for the service, she heard a strange sound coming from one of the children's rooms. She found it odd because no one was staying in that room on this particular weekend. Slowly, she walked over to the door and peaked in. A man lay curled up on the bed, clutching a stuffed bear, sobbing.

Carefully, she backed away without drawing attention to herself. "Hey, Rachel," she said to the nurse that walked by, "who is that in there?"

"It's David's dad."

"What? Really? He came?" David was a boy who had only stayed at Ryan House one time for respite, a stay that occurred a very short time before he went into the hospital for a heart surgery which he did not survive. When David's mother checked him into Ryan House, she explained to Jenni that she and her husband were divorced and that he hardly ever had anything to do with their son.

"He came in and wanted to know which room his son had stayed in. He said he wanted to be in the last place where his little boy was happy."

More and more parents came back to the House for the same reason. Not only do they come to be in the place that made their child so happy, many also want to talk to the staff that knew their child and loved them. Over time, the bereavement counselors discovered parents were far less likely to talk to them since they did not know their children ahead of time. Yet, these same parents frequently opened up to the staff and volunteers at Ryan House.

Sensing an opportunity to provide continuous care, Ryan House started bringing the counselors into the house to interact with the children and their parents ahead of time. They also partnered with a local grief support center and began holding support group sessions at the House for children whose sibling had died. While the children meet all across the house, the parents also sit down and talk through their experiences. Just having the group in the House took these conversations to a whole different level. The House does not close for these group meetings. Children on respite stays still race up and down the halls in their power chairs while a group of moms and dads whose child recently died at Ryan House meet in the Great Room. Something about the sights and sounds of children in the House makes the process of working through grief just a little easier.

Listening to grieving parents opened the door for another change to the original design. The one thing that grieving parents long for is something tangible that connects them to the memories of their child. Meeting that need, Ryan House began providing a Treasured Memories Box. This was inspired by the care that Nancy Flores, then Director of Public Relations and Marketing for Ryan House, and her husband received when their son, Landon, was stillborn after induced labor at seven months. The Treasured Memories Box ensures that each family of a child who has died at the house does not leave Ryan House without special remembrances of their child to treasure forever. Inside, they find a book about grief along with other support materials. In addition, the box contains a homemade pillow that was with the child in the House, along with a model magic casting of the child's handprints and footprints as well as locks of their child's hair, if the family wishes. The Care Team also includes a seed packet and a scrapbook of photographs from the child's time at Ryan House, in addition to written memories from families and friends.

However, parents even wanted more. That's when the idea for the "Story of Me" room arose. The board secured a grant to transform a room with computers into a multimedia, legacy-building room with simple video editing software, along with recording equipment, both audio and video, a green screen, and more. To the children at Ryan House, it's a fun room to go and video themselves telling jokes or playing around with their friends. The grant also provided several Go Pro cameras that children strap onto their wheelchairs for the races through the halls or take with them into the pool as they play there. All the video footage is saved. When a child dies, the Story of Me video becomes one of the parents most treasured possessions.

More changes and adjustments continue to be made the longer Ryan House is open. Some come through the search for better ways to fulfill its original vision. Others are forced on the board and staff as they encounter situations no one has anticipated. Yet none of the growing pains have come as a surprise. Every growing and thriving organization experiences them. And Ryan House continues to be no exception to the rule.

Katie

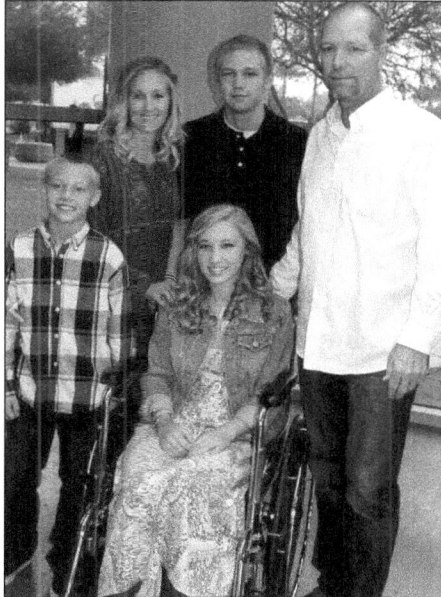

Wagner family

When the oncologists at Phoenix Children's Hospital first mentioned hospice at Ryan House to Steve and Jacque, Katie's mom and dad, Jacque would have none of it. "I don't want to hear that awful word!" she said. "I'm not giving up and hospice means giving up." Steve was more open to the idea but he didn't press the issue. However, when the doctors told them Katie only had a few weeks left, he finally said, "Jacque, we need to at least go and check it out."

"I can't. You go if you want but I'm not going."

"I understand," Steve replied. He went to Ryan House without her, taking along one of his best friends. When he returned he described it with two words: Home and family. She softened a bit. However, she still resisted the idea of needing to take their daughter there any time soon. After all, less than two years earlier she'd been a perfectly normal fifteen year old who loved nothing more than hanging out with her friends. Katie's biggest worry was trying to navigate her way through high school.

Then one day Katie started complaining of stomach pain that would not go away. Doctors thought it was probably a urinary tract infection. Two weeks later the infection remained in spite of treatment. Her doctors decided to do a scope test. That's when they discovered a nine centimeter tumor blocking her bladder. Katie went to school the following Monday while they waited for the results of the biopsy. On Tuesday she was told she had a very rare and very aggressive cancer, Rhabdomyosarcoma, that had already progressed to stage four. She never returned to school.

Over the next seventeen months she received ninety rounds of chemotherapy and over fifty radiation treatments. Six months in, she and her parents were told she was cancer free. The treatments were working. The future looked bright. Then, on her first three month check-up after the last round of chemo, their world came crashing down. The cancer was back, and there was nothing they could do to stop its spread. "We can do more chemo to try to slow it down," the oncologist said, "but it is not a cure. We may be able to add a few months to Katie's life with the treatment."

"I'm not doing any more chemo," Katie said with that firm resolve that told Steve and Jacque nothing they could say would change her mind. That didn't stop them from trying.

"But it may buy you more time," Jacque said.

"My body can't take it. I just can't do it. I just want to live what I have left, hang out with my friends, and be a normal teenager. Is that too much to ask?"

"But, Katie," her mother replied.

"No, mom. Really. I'm okay with this. Besides, my life is in God's hands. If He wants to heal me, He can, with or without more medicine. He healed the blind man without medicine. I think He can do the same for me if it is His will. And if it's not, I know where I am going."

They didn't do any more chemotherapy treatments, although Katie agreed to see a naturopathic doctor for alternative treatments. She did, however, do more than just hang out with her friends.

Before her diagnosis, Katie wanted to go on a mission trip, preferably to Africa. Her cancer made that dream impossible, but she did not give up on the idea of making a difference in the world. Through the organization Water for Our World, she and her friends, Ally and Carly, became aware of a village in Liberia that did not have a school for any of its children. One day while sipping coffee at Starbucks, the three started talking about what they could do to help. "I have a crazy idea," Katie announced. "Let's raise the money ourselves. We can start our own nonprofit and have people donate. Then we can build the school."

Ally and Carly didn't think the idea was crazy at all. The three launched "Stepping Out 4 Hope," with a goal of raising $27,000. They held their first event, a shoe drive, less than a month after Katie's cancer returned. They created their own web page that offered their own merchandise to sell to raise money. People flocked to their Facebook page. Katie had found a way to fulfill her dream without ever leaving Arizona.

But now, less than three months after Stepping Out 4 Hope's first event, Jacque felt she was being asked to give up all hope for her daughter. They brought Katie home from the hospital where they had treated her symptoms, trying to help her breathe. Before they left, Steve and Jacque signed the paperwork for hospice services. Doctors said her time was very short.

Jacque wanted Katie home for as long as possible. However, the cancer had progressed so far that Katie needed around the clock care. A hospice nurse came to the house each day, but only for an hour or two. After one week Jacque knew she could not care for Katie by herself. "I'm ready for Ryan House," she told her husband.

"I think that's the best decision we can make for her," he said. Neither said it at the time but both Steve and Jacque had another reason for moving Katie to Ryan House. They had both finally accepted the inevitability of her situation. They knew they were going to lose their daughter. And both knew they would not be able to walk past her room every day knowing that was where she left this earth.

They called Ryan House and made all the necessary arrange-ments. Dr. Kevin Berger, one of the doctors who works with Ryan House and Hospice of the Valley, had examined Katie and let the staff know her time was very short. He later confided to the fam-ily that he didn't expect her to live through her first night at Ryan House.

Steve and Jacque loaded Katie and some of her favorite things into their car for the drive into Phoenix and Ryan House late Friday afternoon. Brett, her twelve year old brother, could not bring himself to go with them. "I'm going to stay here with Chase," he told them. Chase is Steve and Jacque's oldest son. As Steve backed the car down the driveway, Brett came rushing up on his bicycle. Katie rolled down her window and reached out her hand. Brett couldn't say anything as he took her hand. He sat and sobbed, holding tight onto his sister. "It's okay, Brett," Katie said with a smile. "I will see you again in heaven. I love you." The two sat there for a few moments. Brett just could not let go. Finally, Steve said, "We have to leave."

"Bye, Brett, I love you," Katie said as they drove away.

The Ryan House staff had the room at the farthest end of the hall across from the sanctuary room ready when the family arrived. Jacque wheeled Katie in and said, "This is your room."

"Two beds?" Katie said. "So whose bed is that day bed in the cor-ner? It looks real cozy."

"I know it does, sweetheart, but that's where I'll sleep," Jacque replied. "You need to sleep in the hospital bed so that we can prop you up to help you breathe."

Katie let out a sigh. "That's okay, I guess." That arrangement lasted all of ten minutes. Roni used pillows to prop Katie up in the day bed. Jacque took the adjustable bed. Steve stayed in the family suite across the hall. Halfway through the night, he and Jacque switched places. That way, both would at least get some uninterrupted sleep.

A few days later Katie wanted to see her parent's room. "Wow, this looks really comfortable," she said, then looked over at one of the nurses. "Do you think I..?"

She didn't have to finish her sentence. "Of course you can stay in here if you prefer," the nurse said. "There are no rules here at Ryan House." After that, Jacque and Katie shared the queen sized bed in the family suite. Steve slept in the hospice room. Prior to the move, Katie regularly asked when she could go home. After she settled into her parent's room she was at peace. She never asked to go home again.

What Dr. Berger and others thought would probably be a one or two night stay at the most, turned into thirteen. Brett arrived on the Saturday morning after his sister first came to the House. He never left until the end. Chase went home only to sleep. If he wasn't at work, he was at Ryan House.

It didn't take long for the two brothers to become part of the Ryan House family. Madi, the girl who loves to throw parties, happened to be staying at Ryan House that first weekend. By the end of the day Saturday she had painted both boys' hair at her "Crazy Hair" party. She also took them on wild rides as they held on tight to her power chair as she pulled them down the hallways in an office chair with wheels.

In spite of the fun he appeared to be having, Brett was struggling with what was happening to his sister. He couldn't talk to his parents about what he was feeling. He couldn't talk to anyone. One afternoon Jenni Rogers invited him to join her in the art room. An hour later he came back into Katie's room holding a piece of artwork he'd created. At the top he'd written the words, "Katie is." Then, across the rest of the page he'd pasted words he'd cut out of magazines, each one describing his sister and how he felt about her; words like "indescribable," "kind," and "loving." Jenni took the picture and had it framed for the family. It now hangs in their living room.

The family settled into a routine at Ryan House. Extended family came and went all through the day. A sister-in-law took over the kitchen, cooking not only for Steve, Jacque, Chase, Brett and Katie, but also for the Ryan House staff.

Katie developed her own routine as well. Every morning she wanted to be wheeled to the kitchen for a cup of coffee and a cinnamon roll. In the afternoon she wanted to go to her favorite place at Ryan

House, the oversized bathtub in the bathing room. Whenever she wanted to take a bath, Kasia dropped whatever she was doing and got the room ready. She filled the tub with bubble bath, lowered the lights in the room and put on Katie's favorite music. It took both Kasia and Jacque to get Katie in and out of the tub but neither minded. This was the one place Katie felt most at peace.

Most evenings included a visit from one of the doctors who worked with Ryan House. Several times they told the family that Katie was near the end. Her systems were shutting down. Her ankles swelled, her breathing became even more labored. "She may not make it through the night," they cautioned. Yet, the next morning, Katie would awaken and ask to go to the kitchen for her coffee and cinnamon roll.

One morning, as Jacque wheeled Katie into the kitchen, Katie noticed a baby being pulled down the hall in a red wagon by its mother. "Wait. Stop," she said. "Oh, I want to see the baby. What is her name?" she asked.

The mom pulling the wagon paused, and went over toward Katie. "Her name is Parker," the baby's mother said. Like Katie, Parker was at Ryan House for end-of-life care.

"She is so beautiful," Katie said.

"Thank you," the mom said, her voice cracking.

Later, back in her room, Katie asked her mother, "What was the baby's name again?" The medication her doctors gave her for pain made it difficult for her to remember things as clearly.

"Parker," Jacque replied.

"You mean like a parking lot?" Katie said with an innocent laugh.

"Yes, I suppose so."

"Mom. Would you do me a favor? I need you to go tell Parker's mom not to worry about her. Tell them that I will be in heaven waiting for Parker and I will take care of her until they get there. I know they don't want her to be alone and she won't be. She'll be with me."

Katie's message was a turning point for Parker's mom. She had not been able to turn loose of her child out of fear of who was going to care for her little girl when she died. Knowing Katie was going to be there to welcome Parker home gave her the peace she needed when the time came.

Hanging out with her friends was another big part of Katie's routine. She specifically asked a friend named Diane to come to the House and to bring her guitar. When she arrived, Katie and Diane disappeared into the Story of Me Room for a very long time. Once they finally came back into the room with the rest of the family, Jacque asked, "So what were you two doing that took so long?"

Katie grinned at Diane. "That's a secret."

"Can't you at least give me a hint?"

Katie shook her head. "You'll find out soon enough."

One afternoon toward the end of Katie's stay at Ryan House she decided she needed new glasses. "You need to make me an appointment at Lens Crafters, Mom. I want some new glasses."

"You can't go to Lens Crafters, sweetheart. You are at Ryan House and you can't even breathe."

"But I want new red frames. I'm tired of my old ones."

The conversation went back and forth throughout the day. Finally, Jacque had to put her foot down. "We aren't going to get glasses today. End of story."

Disappointed, Katie did not press the issue. However, a short time later her father mentioned needing to go to the Walgreens just down the street to pick up a few things. "They have glasses at Walgreens, Mom," Katie said. "Can't I please go with Dad?"

Rachel, the nurse who was in the room at the time, overheard the conversation. She looked over at Jacque, shrugged her shoulders and said, "Why not?"

Jacque couldn't believe what she'd just heard. She took Rachel out in the hall and said, "You told me her heart could stop at any moment. How can we possibly go shopping at Walgreens?"

"Listen. It's okay. It's just around the corner. I'll make sure she has plenty of oxygen. If she gets overwhelmed, you can have her right back here in no time."

Jacque reluctantly agreed. After they assembled all the equipment they needed for this short field trip, Steve wheeled Katie to the door and left her there while he went to get the car. Jacque went back to the room to grab one or two more things they might need. While Katie sat there, a volunteer pushed a little girl past in a wheelchair. "My feet are cold," Katie overheard the girl say.

"Bring her over here," Katie said. She then took the little girl's feet in her hands and gently rubbed them. "I hate it when my feet are cold."

"I do, too," the girl said. She looked at the bags sitting next to Katie. "Are you leaving?"

"No. My mom and dad are going to take me to the store."

"That sounds like fun. I love to shop."

"Me, too," Katie said. She sat there, talking with the girl, rubbing her feet, until her dad arrived with the car. "I've got to go now. It was fun talking to you."

"Yeah, me too," the girl said. She grinned as the volunteer wheeled her away. "She's nice," Katie heard her say as her dad wheeled her outside.

When they arrived at Walgreens, Katie tried on every pair of glasses in the store before finally settling on a pair she liked. It was her last shopping trip. Not that she didn't ask to leave for more.

In her last few days the only food she could even think about eating was Cold Stone Creamery ice cream. Going to get some was out of the question, Jacque told her. However, that didn't keep her from having the only food she wanted. Every few days one of the Ryan House staff brought Cold Stone Creamery ice cream into Katie's room for her.

On Thursday morning, September 17th, thirteen days after Katie arrived at Ryan House, she woke up very agitated. "Mom, what is today? What's the special occasion?"

"There's nothing special going on today."

"Yes there is. Is it my birthday? Something's happening. Why are we here?"

"We're at Ryan House and it's just a regular, run of the mill Thursday."

"No, that's not it."

A short time later the nurse Rachel came into the room. "I figured it out," Katie said to her.

"Figured what out? What today is?" Rachel asked.

"Yes! It's a celebration day. It's a celebration for me!"

Rachel looked over at Jacque who mouthed, "I don't know."

"I need to put on makeup today for my celebration," Katie said.

"We don't have any of your makeup here with us but you can use mine if you want," Jacque said.

"Okay." Katie then proceeded to start working on her makeup, but she struggled. A friend, Ally, arrived and helped her. "And I want to wear some cute clothes for my celebration," Katie said. Ally and Jacque helped her change. By the time she finished changing clothes, one of the volunteers stuck her head in the door and said, "You have visitors." Several of Katie's friends had dropped by to see her. They even brought her favorite from Starbucks. Katie didn't have the strength to visit with them for long, but before she left, she went around to each one and said, "Promise me that I will see you again in heaven."

"I promise," one said after another.

"I mean it. You have to keep your promise."

With tears running down their faces, each girl repeated their promise.

"Okay. I have to go, but I will see you again. In heaven. You all promised."

As Jacque wheeled her back to her room, Katie asked, "Mom, was that it?"

"Was that what, sweetheart?"

"Was that my celebration?"

"No baby girl. Your party is waiting for you in heaven and it's much, much better than what we could have done here."

"Okay," Katie replied. She fell asleep when she got back to her room. She slept most of the day. When she was awake, her breathing was even more difficult than normal. Katie became very agitated and afraid. Jacque, Steve, Brett and Chase surrounded her on the queen sized bed in the family suite and calmed her down. They talked, telling her how much they loved her. "I love you, too," she repeated over and over. Amanda, one of the nurses to whom the family had grown very close, came and gave Katie something to help her relax and sleep. Before she drifted off to sleep, everyone said their goodbyes.

"Jacque, Jacque," Jacque heard Amanda say. She had just drifted off to sleep. "You don't want to miss this."

"Steve," Jacque said, awakening her husband. They both looked at Katie. A look of complete peace poured over her face as she took one last breath and stepped over to the celebration waiting for her.

Five months later Katie's friend Diane sent Jacque an email with an audio file attached. "I'm sorry it took me so long to finish this," Diane wrote. "My wedding sort of messed up my schedule. But I wanted to get this just right before I sent it to you. Katie made me promise not to say anything until I'd finished all the editing. I know it will mean a lot to you. It does to me."

Jacque downloaded the audio file and hit play. Katie's voice filled the room singing, "I miss you. I am where I am supposed to be...I am living out my dreams...I know you miss me and I know you miss my face and I miss you."

Stepping Out 4 Hope raised nearly $25,000 for the school in Liberia. The Katie Wagner – Calvary Revival Community School opened there in February, 2014. Jacque, Ally and Carly planned to travel there later that same year. With the school now complete, Stepping Out 4 Hope continues selling t-shirts to raise money for another project Katie loved: Ryan House.

Chapter Thirteen

Just Another Day at Ryan House

THE LAST TIME JASON ARRIVED for his shift as a volunteer at Ryan House, he was more than a little surprised to find Gabriella lying in her bassinet. Today he was not surprised. The hope for a miracle that sprouted in his heart the week before was gone when he saw her. The first time he laid eyes on her he could not believe a child this beautifully alive faced an imminent death. He spent most of his last two weekly volunteer shifts simply sitting and holding her. He was not alone. A long list of volunteers signed up to care for her. Every day someone different held her and loved on her as if she were their own child. Her family rarely came to Ryan House. The shock of her diagnosis and the grim prognosis made it difficult for them to see her. She didn't look like she was dying. If anything, she looked like a typical four-month-old baby girl with a head full of curly, black hair.

"Ready?" Amanda asked as she started to place Gabriella in Jason's arms.

"Of course," Jason said. "This is the best part of my week."

"Prepare yourself because she's had a rough couple of days," Amanda said.

Jason nodded. Even though he was still relatively new at this, he understood the nature of working with the children at Ryan House. During his volunteer training at Hospice of the Valley, the HOV chaplain emphasized the fact that Ryan House wasn't always a happy place with smiling and laughing children with which to play. "Many of the children face end-of-life issues, which is going to be very difficult for you. You will experience very deep grief yourself as you come alongside these children and their families." The chaplain also outlined the grief support services available to both staff and volunteers. Jason didn't give the services much thought at the time. Now he understood how important they are.

Taking Gabriella in his arms, Jason could tell no miracles were in store for her. She labored to breathe and felt even smaller and more frail than he remembered.

"Are you okay? Do you want me to take her?" Amanda asked.

"I'm fine. She's okay right here," Jason replied.

Even though he was single with no children of his own, Jason felt connected to Gabriella from the first time he laid eyes on her. When those big, innocent eyes looked up into his, he was hooked. Each time he held her he could not help but think of how she would never learn to crawl or walk or talk. Yet, as he held her tight, she looked like an angel. Holding her, time seemed to slow down. He became acutely aware of every breath she took, of every small movement her tiny body made. The only thing that seemed to matter was showing this tiny, dying child, how much she was loved and how much her life mattered, no matter how long it might last. "I'm so lucky to get to be here with you, Gabriella," he softly whispered to her as he cradled her in his arms.

Ryan and his buddy, Martine, cruised into the great room in their power chairs to play video games when Brett, the administrative assistant, walked in. "Hey guys, I have a message here that you are needed outside on the playground."

"Really?" Ryan said. "Why?"

"Someone left something out there for you. But first you're supposed to put these on." Brett brought out oversized trash bags for each boy, large enough to cover each boy and his wheelchair.

"Okay, but this seems a little weird," Ryan said.

"Yeah, I'm not so sure about going out for something where I have to wear a garbage bag," Martine added.

"I don't know," Brett said. "I'm just passing on the message I was given."

Since this was Ryan House, both Ryan and Martine knew something was up, but they both played along. They wheeled their plastic covered selves outside to the playground and started looking around. "I don't see anything," Ryan said.

"I think you need to go out a little further, next to the playground equipment," Brett said from just inside the door.

Ryan moved out beyond the patio cover. "You mean here?" he said.

Before Brett could answer, Ryan heard an odd noise. Suddenly, something smacked loudly onto the ground right next to him. Water sprayed up and into his face. He turned to say something to his friend. Before he could get a word out, a red blur flew past, followed by another wet explosion. "WATER BALLOONS!" Ryan yelled. "Take cover!"

Ryan and Martine raced toward the doors under the overhang from the second floor. But before either could get there, another barrage of water balloons blocked their paths. The two boys spun around, laughing hard. "Where..." Ryan said, then he looked up toward the top of the large parking garage immediately north of Ryan House. There, standing on top, was Jim, a Ryan House volunteer who had a reputation for a little mischievous fun. He grinned at Ryan then tossed more balloons down from his perch. Unable to fire any balloons back, since they didn't have any and since it would take a water balloon bazooka to reach the top of a four story structure, the boys darted back and forth across the playground, dodging water balloons and laughing so hard they had to stop from time to time just to catch their breaths.

While the water balloon war raged outside, Julie Bank, Executive Director of Ryan House, met a group from one of the local banks that had scheduled a tour. Julie had met Don, the bank president, four months earlier at the annual Community Breakfast fundraiser held at the Arizona Biltmore Resort. Local community leaders are invited to a free breakfast to learn more about the mission of Ryan House. The program usually consists of a few remarks from Julie followed by a video presentation that highlights life at Ryan House and the families it impacts. It also includes an in-person presentation and testimonial by one of the Ryan House families. Finally, the chairman of the board comes up and makes an "ask."

At the most recent breakfast, Matt Winter, the current board chair, appealed for financial support but also encouraged those in attendance to get involved as volunteers. "It takes two things to keep Ryan House going: treasure and talent," he explained. While the last breakfast netted Ryan House gifts of upwards of $100,000, its greatest value was the list of potential new supporters it supplied the administrative staff.

Today's tour grew out of the last breakfast. Even though Julie is technically off on Saturdays, she often makes an exception for groups like this.
She and Don had talked many times over the past several weeks. The bank
was open to becoming a corporate sponsor for Ryan House. On top of that,
several of their employees wanted to learn more about volunteering. Julie's
experience told her that if even just one or two bank employees got involved
as volunteers and experienced life at the House, Ryan House would capture
their hearts.

Don and four others arrived shortly after noon. "Julie, good to see you
again," Don greeted with a smile as he came in. "Let me introduce you to
everyone." He went through the list of names. Three of his employees were
women and one was a man named Mike who looked to be closing in on
retirement age. Many Ryan House volunteers are retired, including more than
one retired school teacher. The kids really seem to respond to the grandparent
types.

"Let me show you around," Julie offered as she started the tour. "We have
four children staying for respite this weekend and two families for hospice.
I'll show you as much of Ryan House as I can without being too intrusive on
the hospice families or interrupting the fun of the other children." She led
them directly across the hall from the front door into the great room. "This
is our living room. The house is decorated in a camp theme which is why we
call this our Rec Room."

Sponge Bob played on the fifty-inch television. Outside they could hear
Ryan and Martine laughing. A water balloon splashed up against one of the
windows. "That's just a normal day here at Ryan House," Julie explained.

From the "Rec Room" she led them back across the hall into the S'more
Café. Four or five people sat at one table, eating pizza. Julie acknowledged the
group with a "Hi," and then moved on without introducing the tour members
because she knew they were family members visiting an end-of-life child.
She didn't want to impose on their privacy.

Julie then led the group into the art room. Ashley Bogert sat at a table
with a five year old girl. Glitter covered most of the table and part of the floor.

Crayons and markers covered the spots not taken up by the glitter. "This is Ashley, one of our child life specialists," Julie said. She then gave a quick description of the room and what they did there and moved on. While the people on the tour probably thought Ashley was just playing with a child, she was in fact helping her work through some very serious issues, issues with which most adults struggle let alone a five year old. Her cousin was the child at Ryan House for end-of-life care.

Once Julie left, Ashley picked up her conversation with Samantha. "I know your cousin's been here at Ryan House for a few days. Why is he here?"

"He's dying. It's going to look like he's sleeping, but he's not going to be here anymore."

Ashley could tell her parents had tried to explain what was happening to her cousin. However, Samantha is a very bright and perceptive little girl. She asked one question after another which is why her mom and dad asked Ashley to talk with her. They had trouble answering her questions while also dealing with their grief over her cousin dying.

"Do you know why he is dying?" Ashley asked.

"Weeellll, we were going to go swimming, but he started bleeding from his button and that's why he's dying."

Button? What does she mean by button? Then it hit her. He had a G-tube. He'd probably started bleeding from his G-tube which was usually caused by an infection or something like that. Although his bleeding from his G-tube probably had nothing to do with the progression of his disease, in Samantha's mind the two were cause and effect. He was fine until he started bleeding and now he is dying. It all made perfect sense to a five year old.

"Okay," Ashley said. "Let's talk about what's happening with your cousin. Do you know our bodies have some really important parts?"

"Uh huh. I know that," Samantha said as she reached across the table for more glitter.

"The most important part of our body is our brain. Our brain tells the rest of our body what to do. It tells our lungs to breathe. Do you know where your lungs are?"

"I think so," Samantha said.

"They're in our chest. See, put your hand on your chest like this." Ashley put her hand on her chest. Samantha did the same. "Now breathe in and out. Can you feel your chest going up and down?" Samantha giggled. "That's how we breathe. Your cousin has a disease that keeps making it harder and harder for him to breathe. That's why he is dying. His brain keeps telling his lungs to breathe but his lungs are having trouble doing what the brain says. Do you understand?"

"Uh huh."

"Do you have any questions for me?"

"Noooooo, but maybe I will tomorrow."

"Okay, we will talk some more tomorrow. I would like that."

"Yesterday I went to Chuck E. Cheese," Samantha replied. Ashley knew this was a five year old's way of saying she had had enough adult talk for now.

Later, after Samantha finished her picture, she took it and raced down the hall saying, "This is for my cousin who's dying."

Julie's tour stopped to glance in the music room. David, a volunteer who'd retired from teaching a few years earlier, sat at the piano. A teenage boy in a wheelchair was just to one side. Although the boy could not verbally communicate, he smiled wide as David played one chord after another. Julie introduced David to the tour. David, in turn, introduced his friend. "This is Christian and Christian is fourteen and he loves music, don't you buddy?" David said.

"David comes in every other weekend. His wife actually volunteers in our office. She comes in and gets us caught up with a lot of our filing and things like that. But David here loves to work with the kids."

"I sure do. I taught elementary school for, oh my gosh, twenty five years or so. Then I taught teachers at Arizona State. Now I'm here with my buddies like Christian and I'm the one who's being taught."

"What kinds of things do you do here?" one of the tour members asked.

"Whatever they need. I like to be with the kids, but if we're slow around here and they don't need me for that, I'll do anything, work outside on the landscaping, restock the linens, whatever I can do to help. But today I'm playing music with Chris. We're just two old souls who enjoy our time together."

After leaving David and the music room, Julie showed the tour group the "swimmin' hole" and one of the bedrooms that wasn't in use. From there they walked back down toward the other hall. Along the way they passed the reception area. Jason still sat just behind the desk, Gabriella still in his arms.

Julie took the tour group down the short hall to the one family suite that was not in use. "All families are required to stay here with their children the first time they stay for respite. However, we still provide all the care for their children. By having the family stay, it allows an opportunity for them to get to know the care team and help educate them about their child. Care at Ryan House is in place of what families provide at home, so this gives them a chance to show us how they care for their child. We also want the parents to be able to see how well cared for their children are. That gives them the confidence that their kids are in good hands and they will be more likely to feel safe leaving them here with us."

"Do many families stay beyond the first night?" someone asked.

"Some do. Really, some of our best stories come from these rooms. During one couple's first night staying here, the mom walked out in the hallway crying the next morning. Concerned, one of our nurses asked if she could help. The mom told her that this was the first time in three years that she and her husband faced each other in bed. One of them was always with their child. That's why Ryan House is here."

The tour ended in the Memorial Garden. Julie explained the significance of the tiles on the wall and how each stood for a child who had died at Ryan House. Don turned around, scanning each wall. "There are so many," he said.

"Over two hundred fifty now."

"And how long have you been open?"

"Four years."

"That's more than one child a week," Don said, more than a little shocked by the number.

"It is staggering. We have a lot of families who come here for end-of-life care because, before we opened, they really didn't have a child and family-centered place like this where they could go. And when you think about those numbers, the fact that we have two bedrooms for end-of-life care and six bedrooms for respite really puts our care into perspective."

"How often are all eight rooms filled?" someone asked.

"A better question is how often are they not all filled," Julie replied. "Over the past year we've seen tremendous growth in our usage, even though each family is only able to schedule twenty-eight days of respite per year."

"So what can we do to help you, Julie?" Don asked.

"Our biggest need, honestly, is the funding to sustain our operations. We provide all of the services you've seen to families at no charge. Insurance does not reimburse us for respite care, although we do receive some insurance reimbursement for end-of-life care. This year our budget is 2.5 million dollars and we are budgeted to be full to capacity. Our donations range from corporations that give us large grants to ten, twenty, or fifty dollar donations from individuals who believe in what we're doing and want to help. Our fundraising options are pretty diverse and we have opportunities for anyone to get involved. The Kids for Ryan House program offers ideas for kids under 18 to participate, our Professionals Group engages mid-level business leaders. We even have a Grandparents Guild that offers opportunities for anyone who identifies themselves as a grandparent to support our mission. Families are making special memorial donations to honor and remember children who have died at Ryan House. And Ryan House is a qualified charitable organization that donors in our community can designate for their annual "Charitable Tax Credit" (formerly Working Poor Tax Credit) which, as a dollar for dollar return through Arizona, is an easy way to help and can really add up to make a difference.

"You asked what we need and that's the biggest need. My team and I have to constantly raise money so that the people you met today can continue to provide this essential care and Ryan House can continue to support and empower families."

Don nodded. "All right. Anything else?"

"We can always make use of more volunteers who will come in here and love these kids. It's not easy but that's what makes Ryan House, Ryan House. We have a great team of staff and volunteers who make this House a real home. We're always looking for more. We even have opportunities for your bank to volunteer as a group."

Don glanced at his group and smiled, "I think we may want to learn more about both of those."

"Great," Julie said, "I'll keep in touch."

When the group departed, Julie stopped by her office before leaving. She walked past the conference room in the administrative area of the House. A group of high school students was busy making signs for an upcoming fundraising event. Two of the students had siblings who regularly stayed at Ryan House for respite.

On her way out the door, Julie looked over toward the reception area. Jason was passing Gabriella back to Amanda. His shift was over. He leaned over and gave Gabriella a soft kiss on her forehead, his eyes filled with tears. Across the hall, Ryan was back in the living room. He'd been joined by someone Julie recognized as one of the players from the Arizona Rattlers Arena football team. The two were playing a football video game on the television. From the sound of it, Ryan was winning and loving every minute of it.

Julie turned to leave with a smile on her face. This was just another day in the life at Ryan House.

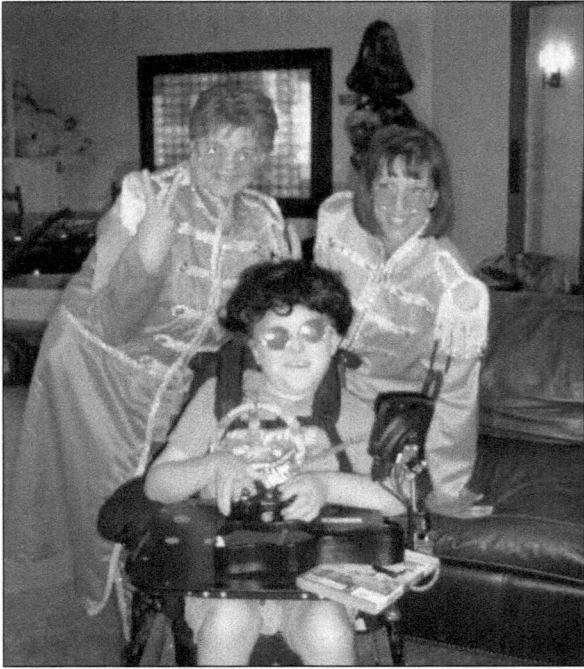

Beatles weekend at Ryan House

Appendix A

WE ARE OFTEN ASKED BY individuals and groups interested in starting this type of care model in their community, "How do we start?" Below were our "strategic goals" from early in our project development that we hope may be useful in creating an action list of what needs to be tackled to help other dreams become a reality.

We wish you all the best of luck…we did it, so can you!

RYAN HOUSE 2004–05 STRATEGIC GOALS
Draft 7.17.04

GOAL 1: COMPLETE FORMAL BUSINESS PLAN

Objective 1: Develop startup and three year operational budget

Strategies

- Study/contact UK, Canadian and US existing House models
- Translate known costs of existing national and international facilities to Arizona dollars
- Determine staffing – paid and volunteers

Objective 2: Secure 501c3 status

Strategies

- Complete necessary documents required for filing
- File IRS 1023 [501(c)(3)] and 557 (tax exemption) documents with Sechler CPA

Objective 3: Create Board of Directors

Strategies:

- Identify and solicit board membership from stakeholder community and steering committee

- Create a medical advisory board
- Create a fundraising task force of the board
- Develop roles and responsibilities

Objective 4: Complete environmental scan (market analysis)

Strategies:

- Examine social, economic, and political trends affecting children with life limiting conditions
- Conduct individual interviews or focus groups of stakeholders including parent groups, physicians, governmental agencies, hospitals and other agencies providing services to children with life threatening conditions
- Perform data analysis
- Write report

Objective 5: Conduct feasibility study to address the revenue sustainability to support ongoing operations

Strategies:

- Hire a consultant to assess currently available 3rd party sources of funds including AHCCCS/Title 19 ALTCS, Division of Developmental Disabilities, Office of Children with Special Health Care Needs, private insurance
- Research Medicaid Waiver via CHI PACC
- Examine other potential revenue streams including community fundraising and fees
- Determine any operational stipulations required, minimum or maximum limits, family implications, and an understanding of how the funds are secured
- Provide recommendations to the Board of Directors

GOAL 2: CREATE PROGRAM SERVICES PLAN

Objective 1: Establish Ryan House within the existing national and international networks of pediatric respite, palliative and hospice organizations to leverage learnings and experiences

Strategies

- Send a representative(s) to one or more of the following conferences

- ARCH National Respite Conference in Atlantic City, New Jersey, September 8-10, 2004

- 16th Annual Children's Hospice International World Congress in Edinburgh, Scotland, September 26-29, 2004

- National Hospice and Palliative Care Organization Conference on Pediatric and Hospice Care in Dearborn, Michigan, November 12-14, 2004

Objective 2: Design program services

Strategies:

- Study/contact UK, Canadian and US existing house models

- Modify program services of existing national and international facilities to Arizona needs

Objective 3: Develop projected three year implementation plan

Strategies:

- Develop phase in model of services to be provided

GOAL 3: CREATE FUNDRAISING PROGRAM

Objective 1: Design and implement a comprehensive fundraising program to support on-going operational costs

Strategies

- Design fundraising plan
- Utilize the Raising More Money® model to initiate a "breakfast kickoff" event, and follow through the fundraising cycle for original point of entry participants
- Secure Customer Relationship Management (CRM) software tools or similar program and determine procedures to efficiently track contacts and actions

Objective 2: Design and implement a capital campaign for Ryan House Facility

Strategies

- Conduct feasibility study
- Determine approach
- Develop fundraising targets
- Implement campaign

GOAL 4: DEVELOP COMMUNITY RELATIONS/MARKETING PLAN

Objective 1: Begin to establish Ryan House within the local Arizona community to raise awareness amongst families with life-limited children, educate the public on the palliative care/hospice model, and build a base for future fundraising

Strategies

- Host a dinner for Valley pediatricians
- Send a representative to the January 14-15, 2005 Governor's Office for Children, Youth and Families conference in Sedona to present Ryan House model as option for families with life-limited children

Objective 2: Create brand for Ryan House

Strategies

- Secure volunteer or paid PR or advertising professional to design branding
- Create collateral materials

Objective 3: Create and maintain a central communication Ryan House website for team and public

Strategies

- Register ryanhouse.org
- Secure a consultant for website set-up
- Create and maintain a calendar of events to be included in website

GOAL 5: CREATE PLAN FOR RYAN HOUSE FACILITY

Objective 1: Evaluate property options and determine site location for Ryan House to focus future planning efforts

Strategies

- Meet with architectural/construction experts to create a preliminary working set of plans that can provide general minimal requirements for the Ryan House (house foundation, parking, garden space, etc.) which can be used to evaluate property options
- Complete a neighborhood assessment for each property option which would subjectively rate issues such as safety, access to off-site activities, noise, zoning restrictions or requirements
- Review any legal and accounting implications

Objective 2: Develop building project budget for the Ryan House facility

Objective 3: Complete timeline for Ryan House launch

The passionate work continues by these amazing people!

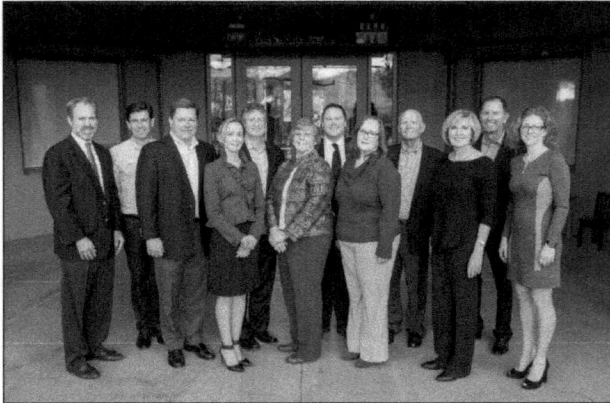

Board of Directors 2015

From left to right: Jonathan Cottor, Dr. Kevin Berger, Matt Winter, Alyssa Crockett, Paul Weiser, Margaret Mullen, Pat Harlan, Janet Moodie, Steve Helm, Leslie Propstra, Eric Butler, Nicole Tarbell

Not pictured: Dr. Kevin Butler, Brady Castro, Rusty Dees, Mary Kirk, Susan Levine, Kate Maynard, Tim O'Neil, Debbie Shumway

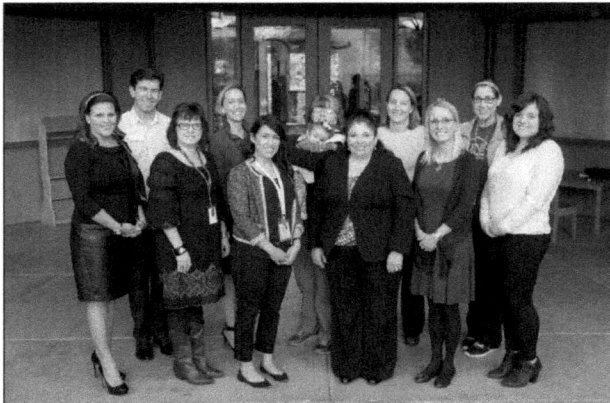

Administrative and Care Team 2015

Back Row: Dr. Kevin Berger, Alyssa Crockett, Kasia Wojnarowska, Dr. Tressia Shaw, Kristen Bakalis

Front Row: Cindy Mero, Pam Roman, Mayda Ramos, Cathy LaSusa, Holly Cottor, Erin Mortensen

Not Pictured: Ashley Kober, Maria Beltran, Nadine Madrid, Grayson Cartwright, Stephanie Moreno, Lucia Collins, Norell Johnson, Dr. Wendy Bernatavicius, Karina Torres, Cesar Tellez

www.ingramcontent.com/pod-product-compliance
Lightning Source LLC
Chambersburg PA
CBHW072125020426
42334CB00018B/1708